THE COMPUTER DIET

A Weight Control Guide

THE COMPUTER DIET

A Weight Control Guide

Vincent W. Antonetti

M. EVANS & COMPANY, INC.
New York, N.Y. 10017

M. Evans and Company titles are distributed in
the United States by the J. B. Lippincott Company,
East Washington Square, Philadelphia, Pa. 19105;
and in Canada by McClelland & Stewart, Ltd.,
25 Hollinger Road, Toronto 374, Ontario

Copyright © 1973 by Vincent W. Antonetti

All rights reserved under International and
Pan American Copyright Conventions

Library of Congress Catalog Card Number: 72-90980
ISBN 0-87131-122-4

9 8 7 6 5 4 3 2 1

To: Rob, Chris, Carrie, Mom and Letty

NOTE

For physicians, nutritionists, dietitians and interested laymen, there is, in Appendix C, a reprint of "The Equations Governing Weight Change in Human Beings," by Mr. Antonetti. This article, which was published by the *American Journal of Clinical Nutrition* in its issue of January 1973, summarizes the research on which Mr. Antonetti based THE COMPUTER DIET.

ACKNOWLEDGMENTS

Many people were involved in the preparation of this book. First I especially want to thank Professor Nicholas A. Carbo of Adelphi University and Mr. Dennis H. Collette, Assistant Administrator for professional affairs at Vassar Brothers Hospital, Poughkeepsie, New York. Both of them took time from their busy schedules to help in so many ways.

For their careful critique of the manuscript, each from the viewpoint of their particular specialty, I want to express my gratitude to: Patricia R. Johnson, Ph.D., physiologist and associate professor at Vassar College; Janet D. Kirk, R.D., dietitian at Vassar Brothers Hospital; Anthony Pietropinto, M.D., Medical Director, Lutheran Medical Center mental health program, New York; Judith S. Stern, D.Sc., assistant professor of nutrition at Rockefeller University; and Norman E. Watt, M.D., of Vassar Brothers Hospital.

I am also indebted to Mr. Rocco J. Budani, vice president of Datatron Processing, Inc., Maspeth, New York and Mr. Bill Williams, data processing manager of the Electronic Tabulating Corporation, Newburgh, New York, for their assistance with the data processing aspects of the book.

Finally, I want to thank Mrs. Joyce Raymond who typed the manuscript.

Author's Preface

My purposes in writing this book are: first, to present the reader with vital new weight control information; and second, to demonstrate the use of this new data in the planning and implementation of a successful weight reduction or weight maintenance program. My approach presupposes a reader with a certain amount of what might be called diet sophistication. I will not, therefore, waste your time with the obvious, and I will not go on, and on, telling you how important it is that you lose weight. In other words, I do not intend to repeat what has been written, over and over again, in every other diet book.

I do hope to provide you with a deeper understanding of weight control and the means with which to approach the problem intelligently. You will be introduced to a great deal of never-before-published data and shown how to use it to your advantage. To do this in the most efficient manner, this book is organized somewhat like a weight control handbook—with the emphasis on facts not frills.

The power of a modern digital computer was used to produce the unique weight control tables which form the heart of this book. Hence, the name *The Computer Diet*. In truth, this book would not have been possible without the many thousands of calculations performed by the computer. Do not, however, let the words "computer diet" mislead you. What follows is not one rigid diet that must be strictly followed, but a multitude of diet options from which you may choose.

It is my hope that dietitians, nutritionists, and medical personnel concerned with weight control will also find the data in this book useful in devising or supervising weight control programs. Whether this book is used as a professional reference, or as a personal weight control guide, my aim is that it will serve the reader as a means to achieving and maintaining a proper weight level.

Contents

Preface	xi
1. Introduction	3
2. Weight and Energetics	11
3. Nutrition and Exercise	17
4. Weight Control: *The Computer Diet Method*	30
5. Weight Loss Calorie Tables	35
6. Weight Loss Diet Tables	104
7. Planning a Weight Loss Program	121
8. Weight Maintenance Calorie Tables	127
9. Weight Maintenance Menu Tables	145
10. Planning a Weight Maintenance Program	212
11. They Did It—You Can Too!	216
Postscript	226
Appendix A. 7-Day Computer Diet	228
Appendix B. Caloric Value of Selected Foods	246
Appendix C. The Equations Governing Weight Change in Human Beings	263
Appendix D. Bibliography	279

Index of Tables

Physical Activity Levels	14
"Ballpark" Calorie Value of Foods	23
Caloric Cost of Physical Activity	25
Desirable Weight	32
Weight Loss Calorie Tables	43
Beverage and Dessert Type Designation	105
Weight Loss Diet Tables	109
Weight Maintenance Calorie Tables	129
Weight Maintenance Menu Tables	147
7-Day Computer Diets	228
Caloric Value of Selected Foods	246

THE COMPUTER DIET

A Weight Control Guide

1. Introduction

"We guarantee a weight loss of two pounds per week," read a newspaper advertisement sponsored by a local weight-control organization. This was about five years ago. My wife wanted to lose ten pounds and decided to attend a "meeting."

Later, as my wife and I discussed what had transpired at the meeting, she said, "There was one point that didn't make sense. When I asked how long I would continue to lose two pounds per week, the speaker answered, 'for as long as you stay on this diet.'"

She laughed when I remarked, "That would mean one year on the diet and you would disappear!"

We both concluded that what must happen in time is that weight loss tapers off. I then asked if the same diet was suggested for everyone. "Yes," she replied, "and everyone is supposed to lose two pounds per week."

I continued, "That really doesn't make sense. In effect, what they are saying is: if you and, for example, Rosey Grier went on the same diet, you would both lose weight at the same rate."

Intuitively, it seemed to me that if my wife and Roosevelt Grier (who is about 6' 6" and probably weighs 260 pounds) were on the same diet, Roosevelt Grier would be practically starving and would certainly lose more weight than would my wife.

At that time, I had stopped smoking and had promptly gained ten pounds. I was still gaining when I joined the

YMCA. The exercise made me feel more vigorous and fit, but I had not changed my eating habits, and I didn't lose weight.

As I recall, it was that conversation with my wife, and my own inability to lose weight, that first aroused my interest in weight control. Over the next five years, this casual interest grew into a research project, which included a literature search, a mathematical analysis, publication of a scientific paper, and most recently, this book.

Research

I began by reading every popular diet book I could find. Frankly, I was not satisfied. The books were contradictory, and perhaps because I am an engineer, I found they lacked the kind of quantitative information I was looking for. I gravitated toward scientific literature. I read books on physiology, nutrition, and then, the latest pertinent research papers. I began to correspond with scientists at leading universities.

From my literature search, I found a tremendous amount of on-going weight control research. I learned that there are two fundamentally different schools of thought concerning the nature of weight loss. One view argues that "calories-do-count," or in more scientific terminology, that weight loss is governed by the law of conservation of energy (which will be discussed in greater detail in Chapter 2). The contrary view is that certain foods or food combinations have special qualities that cause weight to be lost more rapidly than would be predicted by the law of conservation of energy. I appraised the evidence on both sides, and the more deeply I read, the more convinced I became that the "calories-do-count" group was right. It seemed perfectly reasonable to me that the human metabolism should obey the law of conservation of energy—as does everything else in nature!

I further reasoned that if the law of conservation of energy does apply to the human metabolism, it should be possible to do a mathematical analysis of weight change in human beings. For years, researchers have recognized that such weight change is a function of— at the very least—age, sex, height, weight, amount of physical activity, caloric intake, and time. Unfortunately, the relationship of these factors to weight change had never been mathematically established. With the background I had acquired in physiology and nutrition, plus my engineering-mathematics training and experience, I set myself the task of developing the formulas involved in weight change.

Engineering and Weight Control

That I would attempt such an analysis is not as unusual as it might appear. The reader should be aware of the existence of a relatively large group of engineers working in a field that falls somewhere between medicine and engineering, called bio-medical engineering. For years, these engineers have been developing advanced technology for use in medicine. Applications of engineering to medicine range from the development of cryogenic surgical instruments and electronic surveillance systems for hospitals to the development of prototype mechanical hearts. Engineers have also devised mathematical models of various parts of the human body in order to analyze and, therefore, better understand their function. Such analyses include the application of engineering control theory to the function of the human brain and utilization of the laws of fluid mechanics to study the blood circulatory system. Moreover, any significant understanding of weight control requires a knowledge of the first law of thermodynamics as applied to the human metabolism. Therefore, my particular engineering specialties, which are thermodynamics and heat transfer, are especially suited to this kind of research.

Many of my friends were openly skeptical. "You can't do that. You can't analyze the human body as if it were a machine!" My response was that the human body is a machine. The most complex and challenging machine I had ever worked on. But I was sure that by taking the proper analytical approach, the equations could be derived.

The Weight Change Equations

The method of analysis I employed was not new. Engineers call the technique a generalized closed system approach. It has been used to solve many fundamental thermodynamic problems. In simple terms, the analysis is performed by considering the human body as a closed system, and observing what forms of energy and mass cross the system's boundaries. In this method, one is not concerned with what is happening inside the closed system (body). Only external energy and mass transformations are of importance; once identified, these external quantities are then related in accordance with the law of conservation of energy. As an analogy: the performance of a large and complex chemical process plant, with its maze of piping and equipment, can be understood and predicted by writing the equations relating the energy and mass of the various chemical streams entering and leaving the plant—without considering the internal reactions.

In the course of the development of the weight control equations, certain physical, biological, medical, and nutritional data were needed. In all cases, I obtained this information from the latest and best scientific sources.

The weight control equations I developed represent a mathematical model of one facet of the human metabolism and provide a means to answer questions such as: How long will it take an individual of a given sex, age, height, weight, and activity level to lose a desired amount of weight when on a known diet? And, how should one adjust his diet to maintain this new weight?

The Minnesota Experiment

Once the weight change equations were derived, the next step was to validate that they did indeed accurately predict weight change. There are essentially two ways to accomplish this. The first method involves setting-up a series of experiments in order to observe the weight loss of various subjects. This technique would necessitate a research facility and would take years to accomplish. The second method is to compare the theoretical predictions of the equations, against weight loss data gathered over the years by various research teams. Of course, I decided on the latter technique.

Although there is a great deal of weight loss data in the medical literature, the most famous and comprehensive collection of data was gathered during what became known as The Minnesota Experiment. The timeframe of the experiment was near the end of World War II. A team of research scientists at the Laboratory of Physiological Hygiene at the University of Minnesota had received reports that starvation was present in the occupied areas of Europe and in the prison camps. There was a danger of mass famine. It was evident that at the end of hostilities the United States would be involved in a large-scale nutritional program. They recognized that what was required, immediately, was an experiment to determine what changes occurred in man due to semi-starvation and what would be the best kind of rehabilitation diet.

The subjects for the experiment were a volunteer group of conscientious objectors, who welcomed the opportunity to serve as human guinea pigs. The men were put on diets of approximately 1500 calories per day for six months and then, of course, they were renourished. The data collected from the experiment is documented in a two-volume treatise entitled *The Biology of Human Starvation*. Among the myriad data gathered during the study was a tremendous amount of carefully recorded weight loss information. I analyzed this data and found that my weight change equations predicted the weight loss experienced by the conscientious objectors quite well.

I did not stop checking. I compared the predictions of my weight change equations against other well-documented experiments conducted by research laboratories on obese patients. In a variety of tests, patients were subjected to all types of diets—high-fat, high-protein, low-carbohydrate, and so forth. As I suspected, the type of food eaten did not significantly alter the weight loss prediction. For a given subject, only the number of calories consumed appeared to be important. Now satisfied, I wrote a paper documenting my research.

A Scientific Paper

The article, "The Equations Governing Weight Change in Human Beings," which was published by the *American Journal of Clinical Nutrition,* reports the results of my research. In the article, the disciplines of engineering and physiology are united to establish the foundation for a truly rational approach to weight control for human beings.

"Appears quite logical and straightforward," said a chemist friend, after I showed him my paper. "But," he continued, "it is not going to be used. The average medical doctor or dietitian is not sufficiently skilled in mathematics to be able to apply your equations in practical weight control situations. Unless you translate your equations into a more practical form, you have wasted your time!"

The Weight Control Tables

My friend was right. The weight change equations I developed are relatively complex. One would have to be proficient in advanced mathematics to apply the equations to a particular individual on a given diet. Tables, I thought, might be the answer. In tabular form the equations would be useful. Devising a tabular format was almost second nature to me. As a matter of fact, my colleagues often kid me because of my tendency to automatically arrange virtually any set of information into a table. As you read on you will know what they mean. In a short time, however, I realized that it would take me years to do the calculations needed to produce the tables I had in mind. To compute just one number in the table took more than half an hour, and there were thousands of numbers to calculate! Twenty years ago, this would have meant the end of my project, but with the advent of the modern digital computer, calculations of this scope are commonplace. Therefore, I proceeded to program the weight control equations. Using a digital computer I reduced them to a series of easy-to-use weight control tables, published for the first time in this book. These unique tables make it possible for anyone to quickly determine the exact caloric intake (diet) necessary to lose a given amount of weight or to maintain a desired weight level.

The Computer Diet Approach

In the following chapters, the reader will first be introduced to the relationship between weight control and energy. Next will follow a "cram course" in the basics of sensible nutrition and exercise. Then the heart of the book: the unique weight loss and weight maintenance calorie, diet, and menu tables which provide the basis for the computer diet. The use of these valuable new tools in the development of a *logical and personalized* weight control plan will be described in detail. In addition, the Appendix includes 7-day reducing diets of 900, 1200, 1500, 1800 and 2100 calories per day, a caloric value table, and a comprehensive bibliography.

2. Weight and Energetics

Conservation of Energy in the Human Body
All human life depends on energy. The sun's energy is used by plants to make food, and man uses the energy found in food to operate his body. One of the greatest achievements of the nineteenth century was the recognition and statement of the principle of conservation of energy by Julius Robert Von Mayer, in a classic paper that appeared in 1842 in Liebig's *Annalen der Chemie*. The principle is an inductive generalization based on the observation of physical phenomena. The law of conservation of energy states that energy may be converted or transferred, but cannot be created or destroyed. Von Helmholtz, a surgeon in the Prussian army, recognized the importance of this principle, and in 1847 wrote a brilliant paper applying the idea to the sciences of physiology and chemistry. By the beginning of the twentieth century, the scientific observations of Rubner, and then of Atwater and Benedict, had demonstrated the validity of the law of conservation of energy for the human metabolism.

According to the law of conservation of energy—as related to the human organism—the energy value of the food eaten (minus the energy lost in the excreta) must equal the sum of the heat given off and the physical work done by the body. Most scientists today agree that weight change in human beings is related to their energy imbalance and, in fact, weight loss is in accordance with the law of conservation of energy.

The unit of measure of heat energy is the calorie. Both the energy value of the food we eat and the energy we expend in day-to-day activity are expressed in terms of the calorie.

When Weight Change Occurs

Simply stated, the generally accepted theory is that weight loss in human beings occurs when the energy expended by the body is *greater* than the energy value of the food consumed. An energy imbalance is present when this condition exists. In order to return to a state of energy balance, the body compensates by "burning" stores of body weight—mainly adipose tissue—which results in the liberation of available energy. The net result of this process is a loss in body weight and a return of the body to an energy balance or equilibrium, in accord with the law of conservation of energy. The process of weight gain can be explained by applying the converse of this reasoning.

Total Energy Requirements of the Body

Since body weight is only lost or gained during an energy imbalance, there is no weight change when the energy value of the food consumed equals the amount of energy required by the body to maintain its present weight. How much energy does a human being need? To answer this question, one must be aware of the energy constituents that comprise the body's total needs. The energy requirement of human beings is made up of four parts: 1. Basal metabolic energy, 2. Activity energy, 3. Ingestive energy, 4. Energy required for growth.

Weight and Energetics 13

This book is confined to a discussion of the weight control needs of adults, and therefore only the first three types of energy will be discussed.

Basal Metabolic Energy

The basal metabolic energy is that energy which is expended in performing the body's basal processes. These basal functions are involuntary and include circulation, respiration, glandular activity, operation of the kidneys, and the contractions of the intestines, etc. All of these processes consume energy. Scientists determine the basal energy by a very carefully controlled test in which measurements are made on a subject while he lies quietly and completely relaxed. The results of this kind of test show that the basal metabolic energy is dependent on sex, age, height, and weight, and that most individuals vary within plus and minus ten percent of what is considered normal.

Activity Energy and Activity Levels

As soon as one begins to move about, the physical activity causes energy expenditure to increase significantly above the basal level. Many experiments have been performed to determine the energy equivalent of various types of activity; the results are usually listed in terms of calories per pound per unit of time. Thus to compute one's total energy requirement due to physical activity, a diary of the amount of time spent at each activity should be kept for an entire day; the total activity energy expended for the day would then be calculated by multiplying the amount of time spent at each activity by the caloric value per unit of time for each activity. Obviously, such a detailed determination would in most cases be impractical; because of this I have developed a new and more accessible measurement called the Activity Level for your use. Essentially, to use the Activity Level method, you must make a judgment of your physical activity energy expenditure. Admittedly, this is the least quantitative section of this book because it depends on a subjective assessment by the individual. Nevertheless, I feel that the approach advocated here is the most workable in practical, day-to-day situations. The various levels are defined in the table headed Phys-

PHYSICAL ACTIVITY LEVELS

ACTIVITY LEVEL	NAME	DESCRIPTION
0	Sedentary	Inactive most of the day. Very little standing or walking.
1	Light	Seated a major portion of the day. About four hours of standing and walking. Typical of the office worker and those with similar occupations.
2	Moderate	Stands as often as is seated. Typical of the teacher, young housewife, sales clerk, etc.
3	Vigorous	Standing and walking most of the day. Very little sitting. Typical of the factory worker, farmer, construction worker, etc.
4	Severe	Very hard physical work. Typical of the lumberjack or athlete in training.

ical Activity Levels. To determine your Activity Level will, in most cases, require considerable judgment. For instance, all housewives are not necessarily in category 2. The mother of three youngsters under four years of age may lead quite a hectic life and might very well qualify for Activity Level 3. On the other hand, a housewife with no children at home and only a small apartment to care for might more accurately belong in the first category. It should be kept in mind that modern technology has reduced physical demands, and that most people today are not as active as their ancestors and, therefore, require lower calorie allowances. In fact, the typical American female probably belongs in Activity Level 1, while the average male is between Activity Levels 1 and 2. Once you determine your Activity Level, you are ready to use the Weight Loss and Weight Maintenance Calorie Tables in Chapters 5 and 8.

Ingestive Energy

In a classic experiment in calorimetry, the famous French scientist Lavoisier discovered that the ingestion of food caused an increase in the heat produced by the body. This increase is due to the physical work involved in the mastication, digestion, and elimination of food. This process is called the influence of food or specific dynamic action. Ingestive energy was taken into account in deriving the equations and tables used in this book.

Another factor which influences the amount of energy expended by the body is the ambient or environmental temperature. Ambient temperature is of negligible importance, however, to energy expenditure in temperate zones where people are well-clothed and houses are well-heated, and was therefore not considered.

Calories or Carbohydrates?

Every so often a low carbohydrate fad diet becomes popular and its adherents monitor the amount of carbohydrate grams they consume. You will notice that in the preceding discussion of weight control and energetics I made no special point regarding carbohydrates. This is because eating too many calories will result in a weight gain, whether the nutrient the calories are from is protein, fat, or carbohydrate. As stated previously, weight change is governed by the law of conservation of energy, and the measure of energy is the calorie. So calories count, and counting carbohydrate grams is pure nonsense!

3. Nutrition and Exercise

Proper weight is only one facet of total health. There are other equally important requirements. It is generally agreed that a high level of well-being is achieved when this proper weight is the result of a total program based on sound nutritional practices and a good exercise routine. In the chapters on weight loss and weight maintenance that follow, you will be shown how your food intake and energy expenditure affect your weight. But first, you should understand what nutritional guidelines to follow in establishing your food intake and what methods of energy expenditure are particularly conducive to total physical fitness. This chapter, however, is not a dissertation on nutrition or physical education; rather, it might more accurately be described as a cram course designed to allow you to apply the basics of nutrition and exercise to the development of a well-rounded weight control plan.

Essential Food Groups

A normal person will generally eat at least an amount of food necessary to satisfy his energy requirements. Surveys of the diets of adults, however, show that many people choose foods that fail to supply an adequate amount of nutrition. For this reason, the concept of Essential Food Groups was developed some years ago as a means of setting nutritional guidelines in food selection. The theory is that many foods are similar in their nutritional properties and therefore can be thought of as part of the same group of foods. According to the U.S. Department of Agriculture, there are four broad Essential Food Groups: 1. Milk Products, 2. Meat Group, 3. Fruits and Vegetables, 4. Bread-Cereals Group.

Milk Products: Includes skim milk, cheese, yogurt, etc. Many nutritionists consider milk to be the best all-around food, with the greatest assortment of nutrients. It is high in complete protein and calcium. At least two portions per day are recommended for adults.

Meat Group: Includes poultry, fish, eggs, dried legumes, and nuts. Meat, poultry, fish, and eggs are excellent sources of high-quality complete protein, while nuts and dried legumes, although of lower nutritional quality, are inexpensive alternates. At least two servings per day are recommended from this group.

Fruits and Vegetables: These are important sources of vitamins and minerals. For vitamin A, you should eat a dark-green or one deep-yellow vegetable at least every other day. Have either a citrus fruit or other vitamin C-rich fruit or vegetable (such as oranges, grapefruit, strawberries, or tomatoes) daily. In addition, choose two more servings of any other fresh fruit or vegetable every day.

Bread-Cereals Group: Includes whole grain cereals, bread, rice, noodles, and so forth. They are good sources of vitamin B-complex and iron. Four servings per day are recommended unless in doing so you exceed your caloric allowance.

You should strive to eat at least the amounts recommended from each of the essential food groups. Some fat (particularly in the form of vegetable oil) should also be included in your diet. Variety in selection is very important, from both the nutritive and diet interest viewpoints.

Prudent Nutrition

Of late, researchers have written a great deal linking high levels of serum cholesterol with coronary heart disease. With this in mind, it would seem prudent particularly for men, and women past menopause, to restrict their intake of dietary cholesterol and saturated fats. These persons should limit themselves to two visible eggs per week. They should also reduce the amount of butter they use, drink skim milk in place of whole milk, substitute fish and poultry for meat as often as possible, and cut down on the amount of rich desserts they consume.

Because young women of childbearing age rarely suffer from coronary heart disease, they need not be as concerned about these matters. Most nutritionists, however, advocate that men and women of all ages reduce their intake of sugar in its various forms.

Allocating the Day's Calories

Current nutritional theory suggests a meal pattern that features frequent small meals and a fairly even distribution of the daily caloric allowance over the day's meals —whether you are on a reducing or a weight-maintenance type of diet. Most people, however, eat three meals a day, and in most instances it would probably be impractical to increase the number of formal meals. Ideally, what I would recommend is that you eliminate some food from each formal meal and add three nutritious snacks to your daily eating routine. A practical rule of thumb for allocating the day's calories is as follows: Divide your total daily caloric allowance equally among breakfast, lunch, dinner, and your collective in-between-meal snacks. In later chapters, you will be shown how to determine your daily caloric allowance. For now, let us assume it amounts to 2400 calories. Using my rule of thumb, you divide 2400 by 4 and find you should allot 600 calories for each of your three main meals and save 600 for between-meal snacks. Assuming you decide on three snacks, your daily caloric split would be: 600 for breakfast, 600 for lunch, 600 for dinner, and 200 calories each for three snacks.

This example represents an ideal calorie distribution. Your aim should be to get as close to the ideal as you can, but make sure the eating pattern you establish is one you can realistically follow. By habit, the average person is likely to eat a relatively light breakfast, a moderate lunch, a heavy dinner, and perhaps one snack per day. Not exactly the ideal, but I would not suggest a drastic change at the start. Begin with a compromise. For instance, the 2400 calories from the previous illustration might be split as: 500 calories each for breakfast and lunch, 1200 calories for dinner, and 200 for a snack. Whatever your allocation, by all means do not skip a meal. Do set a regular calorie distribution system that you can live with, and give yourself time to adjust to the ideal.

Meal Patterns

Start with a good breakfast! How often you must have heard that. You should realize that the statement is valid even when you are on a reducing diet. After the night's fast, your body needs food energy to accomplish the morning's work. A good breakfast should begin with an unsweetened juice or a fresh fruit that is high in vitamin C, and for young women should be based on protein foods such as skim milk and eggs. Men (and women past menopause) should have cereal and skim milk, or perhaps cottage cheese. This type of breakfast will provide a feeling of satiety and well-being that will last until lunch. Incidentally, you should be hungry when you awake in the morning. If you are not, you probably overate the night before.

A well-balanced lunch need not be elaborate. As with all the day's meals, the primary ingredient should be some type of protein food. You should also try to include a green salad and fresh fruit for dessert in your luncheon menu.

Dinner is traditionally the main meal of the day and should be planned around meat, poultry, or fish. Cheese, eggs, or legumes may be substituted occasionally. You should have a dark-green leafy or deep-yellow vegetable with this meal, if it has not been served earlier in the day.

Caloric Value of Foods

You must be able to judge the caloric value of foods if you are going to successfully control your weight. To my way of thinking, the procedure involved in determining the caloric content of a meal is somewhat analogous to solving an engineering problem. For this reason, it will be to your advantage to use an engineering-like approach.

The first thing an engineer does when performing a design calculation is to "ballpark" his answer. You will often hear an engineer remark, "Should that gidget be one or ten inches thick? What ballpark are we in?" Initially, he performs a relatively crude, quick, and usually over-simplified calculation which "ballparks" his answer. Next, time and circumstances permitting, he goes back and does a more thorough analysis, considering all the subtleties of the problem. I recommend that you approach calorie counting in much the same manner.

For example: you are having dinner at a friend's home, and you are served a great-tasting concoction you hardly recognize. You know you are going to overeat. So you try to make a mental estimate of the calorie content of the meal—in that way you can compensate the next day. Naturally, you don't have access to an accurate calorie chart, and even with one (without knowing the exact ingredients of the recipe) you would probably be lucky to come within 50 calories of the true total. In this situation, don't waste your time trying to decide if you should use a value of 65 or 70 calories for that piece of bread you just ate, when your best guess on the main dish is a number between 400 and 600 calories. What you should do in this situation is "ballpark" your answer.

To "ballpark," you first should know what elements are significant in the calculation and then what approximate values you should assign to these elements. In other words, you should know what foods you should even bother counting and then what approximate caloric value you should give these foods. The table called "Ballpark" Caloric Value of Foods is designed to help you make quick and reasonable estimates. The values in the table are purposely rounded-off to make them easier to memorize and use. And I do suggest you memorize the values in the table.

Of course, when the situation permits a more accurate calculation, you should do so. In such cases, refer to the comprehensive tables labeled Caloric Value of Selected Foods, which appear in Appendix B.

"BALLPARK" CALORIC VALUE OF FOODS

BREAKFAST
Juice (small)	50
Cereal and milk (bowl)	200
Egg (any style)	100
Bacon slice	50
Toast, buttered	100
Coffee, black	0
Coffee, regular	50
Pancake	100
Syrup (Tbsp.)	50
Butter (pat)	50

LUNCH AND DINNER
Soup (1 cup, water base)	100
Soup (1 cup, milk base)	200
Sandwich	400
Cottage cheese (1 cup)	250
Hard Cheese (1 oz.)	100
Fish (1 oz.)	40
Lean meat, poultry (1 oz.)	60
"Regular" meat (1 oz.)	80
Gravy (Tbsp.)	50
Potato	100
French Fries	150
Green salad	0
Salad dressing (Tbsp.)	100
Vegetables (1 cup)	100
Stew (1 cup)	250
Spaghetti and meat balls	500
Bread	75

BEVERAGES
Skim milk (1 cup)	100
Wine (small glass)	100
Beer (can)	150
Soda (can)	150
Hi-ball	150

DESSERTS
Fruit	50
Cookie	50
Donut	125

"BALLPARK" CALORIC VALUE OF FOODS

Cake (plain)	200
Ice cream (1 cup)	250
Pie	350
Cheese cake	350

Judging Portion Sizes

Another dilemma for dieters is judging portion size. It doesn't make sense to worry about whether to allocate 60 or 70 calories per ounce for lean meat if you have no idea whether the slice of meat you are about to eat weighs four or ten ounces. Learn to judge portion sizes with reasonable accuracy. The best way to do this is to start by carefully weighing and measuring the food you eat. After about a week, your eye should be adjusted to what four ounces of meat looks like, and you can then discontinue the weighing routine. Incidentally, judging the weight of meat is one of the most important parts of a diet. As a guide, four ounces of meat would be roughly about 4 x 4 x ¼ inch in size (the size of a slice of white bread). Calorie tables always refer to meat that has been cooked and trimmed of fat and bone. Make sure you allow for these points.

Exercise Fundamentals

Because exercise requires energy expenditure, it tends to cause an energy deficit and helps to accelerate weight loss. It is not usually practical, however, to count on exercise as the sole means of losing weight. This is because of the relatively low caloric cost of even a very strenuous workout. The table labeled Caloric Cost of Physical Activity shows, for instance, that if you weigh 150 pounds and run at the very fast rate of 10 mph you-will expend 960 calories in one hour. After six minutes at this pace, you will have covered one mile and burned all of 96 (960 ÷ 10) calories! If it is at all comforting, the heavier you are the more calories you expend during exercise. For example, if you weigh 210 pounds and ran along with the 150-pounder, after one mile you would have burned 135 calories!

CALORIC COST OF PHYSICAL ACTIVITY

TYPE OF ACTIVITY	BODY WEIGHT—lbs.					
	120	150	180	210	240	270
Lying still	6	7	8	10	11	12
Sitting quietly	22	27	32	39	44	49
Standing	27	35	41	48	54	60
Ironing clothes	54	66	84	96	108	120
Walking (3 mph)	108	138	162	192	216	246
Carpentry	126	156	186	222	252	272
Cycling (moderate)	138	168	204	240	276	306
Dancing	162	204	246	288	324	365
Walking (4 mph)	187	229	277	324	374	414
Skating	192	240	288	336	384	427
Sawing wood	312	384	453	547	624	697
Swimming (2 mph)	426	533	642	758	852	968
Boxing	619	775	930	1085	1238	1390
Running (10 mph)	770	960	1160	1350	1540	1740
Rowing in race	870	1090	1300	1520	1740	1960

Values in table: calories expended for one hour of activity (above basal metabolic level).

Nevertheless, exercise is important to total well-being and should be a part of everyone's daily routine. It tones the muscles, improves the circulation and the operation of the heart and lungs. Two types of basic exercise are of special interest: the muscle-building type and the aerobic type. The muscle-building type includes calisthenics and weightlifting. The aerobic exercises are those that force one to breathe deeply, and include jogging, running, cycling, and swimming. The muscle-building exercises increase strength, agility, and coordination. The aerobic type primarily exercise the heart, lungs, and circulatory system. While most physical fitness experts recommend both kinds of exercise, the majority agree that for the average person the aerobic type are an absolute necessity for real well-being.

To be safe, an exercise routine should be supervised by a physician and should start with a medical examination. According to Dr. Kenneth Cooper, a recognized authority on physical fitness, a good exercise program should progress slowly toward more rigorous exercise. It should consist of aerobic exercises done regularly. The participant should take care to warm up properly, always exercise within his tolerance, and cool down slowly.

An Engineer's Approach to Physical Fitness

My personal physical fitness program started about five years ago. As I have already mentioned, I had decided to stop smoking—after sixteen years. When I began to gain weight, I started on an exercise routine, but still could not lose weight. At 5′ 9″ and 175 pounds, I was at least twenty pounds over my ideal weight.

At this point, I did not yet appreciate the mathematics involved in weight control but I had acquired an understanding of the basics of nutrition. With the help of a dietitian friend, I devised a well-balanced 2100 calorie diet (very similar to that shown on page 244). I also made an important decision. I decided to adjust the priorities in my life so that physical fitness was second only to my family. In summary, then, my personal physical fitness program consisted of a 2100 calorie reducing diet, an exercise routine in which jogging was the main activity, and, of course, I stopped smoking.

Some authorities say you should not attempt all of these at once because of the total self-discipline required for success. I do not agree. All three of these fitness aspects are related. I found that the will power required to adhere to my exercise program was akin to that needed for my diet, and that success in one phase actually reinforced my total determination. For example, after an exhilarating workout I would feel fantastic, and I could not think of smoking or eating and negating any good I had just accomplished.

I began by getting a medical check-up, and when my physician gave me his approval, I started a jogging routine. At first I could not run a mile without stopping several times to rest. (The tendency is to run too fast in the beginning.) After a month of running relatively short distances, walking long distances, and doing calisthenics, I could actually feel a general improvement in my condition. It was then that I tried to jog a full mile. A friend set a very slow pace, and I completed the mile in 10 minutes and 30 seconds. I was exhausted, but I had made a mile!

From that point on, I very slowly and carefully quickened my pace, week by week. Depending on how I felt, I would jog one to three miles one day and exercise with weights the next. As my training program progressed, the aches and pains disappeared, and I can still remember the sensation of well-being I experienced at the end of each session. Returning home from the gym I would fill my lungs with the night air, and I felt I could breathe more deeply than I ever had thought possible. I could feel every muscle in my body, and although I knew I had only burned 200 to 300 calories—I actually felt slimmer! Most certainly this feeling gave me a mental boost that helped me through the other parts of my program.

I ran at the YMCA and followed custom by recording my time and distance on the bulletin board at the end of each session. I was so proud of my progress that I would post my time for the mile on a graph at work. In five weeks my time dropped to less than 8 minutes for one mile.

Mid-way in my conditioning program I completed the derivation of my weight change equations. Anxious to try them out, I used myself as the subject of an experiment. I had been keeping a diary of my daily caloric intake and body weight. (I weighed myself every Wednesday night at the same time, on the same scale, and in the same state of undress.) To my delight my weight dropped precisely as the equations predicted.

One hundred days from the start of my serious training and dieting, I had achieved my ideal weight, I was running two miles in less than 15 minutes, and I was quite sure I had the cigarette habit beaten!

Having achieved my goals, I adjusted my calorie intake upward to 2850 calories per day. (You will learn, on page 133, that this is the maintenance calorie value for a male between 18–35 years, 5' 6" to 5' 11" tall at Activity Level 2.) I also decided to change my workout so that I now run approximately 2 miles per day and I no longer monitor my time for the distance. My reasoning is that there are enough deadlines to meet in modern life, and once you are in reasonably good condition, there is no need to associate time with your workout. I let my body chemistry decide how fast I will run on any particular day. But I continue to monitor my diet.

Some five years have passed since I first started my physical fitness program and I still weigh 155 pounds. I have observed many people who have lost weight on a variety of programs, but I know of very few who have maintained their lower weight level. Why? In my opinion, successful weight control over a period of years comes to those who have some degree of self-discipline and to those who know what they are doing. You have to know what you are doing to succeed at weight control! That is why this book is valuable. Read on!

4. Weight Control: The Computer Diet Method

Why Are You Overweight?

I am going to assume that you have consulted with your physician and have no physiological disorder (glandular, digestive, etc.) which would prevent you from losing weight. Very few people are obese because of these reasons.

Back to the question posed. Once you accept the fact that the law of conservation of energy applies to the human metabolism, the answer is simple enough. You are overweight because you consume more calories than you expend. Inactivity or overeating, or a combination of both, are the culprits. They are, however, the cause of your weight gain, not the reason for it.

The question might more properly be: Why do you eat more than you should? Scientists offer two fundamentally different opinions. On the one hand, it is thought that the body's metabolism is at fault. There may be some subtle metabolic, regulatory, or developmental disorder which affects hunger-satiety signals and, in effect, causes a person not to know when to stop eating. On the other hand, it is proposed that the problem is more behavioral in nature. In other words, overeating may be associated with neurosis or other psychological problems.

The fact is that although you may never understand

the underlying cause for your being overweight, you can still lose weight successfully by understanding and applying the basics of sound diet theory.

What You Should Weigh

Among the methods of assessing whether an individual is at the proper weight level are: the mirror test, the ruler test, the belt line test, the measurement of skin-fold thickness, and the measurement of total body water. Some of these are very subjective; others are too scientific to be practical for the layman. For these reasons, the Desirable Weight chart, although far from perfect, is still probably the most popular means. To use the chart in this book, you will have to assess your frame size. One simple way to do this is to compare the size of your wrist with that of others of the same sex and height. Is it large by comparison? If so, you probably have a large frame.

Computer Diet Weight Loss Program

You have probably tried almost every type of diet—crash, pills, water, grapefruit, high-protein, low-carbohydrate, whatever. I think you will agree that a typical shortcoming of these popular quick-weight-loss diets is that they lack quantitative data. In addition, many of these fads are neither medically nor scientifically oriented nor do they contain factual or reliable information. Yes, the computer diet is different!

How? First, I believe it is the most logical and scientifically sound diet you will ever use. (You will be shown exactly what to do and told why.) Next, the diet is based on the latest available quantitative information. (By using the Weight Loss Calorie and Diet Tables that follow, your understanding will be such that *you* will be

DESIRABLE WEIGHT

HEIGHT (without shoes)	WEIGHT (without clothing)		
	SMALL FRAME	MEDIUM FRAME	LARGE FRAME
Men	Lbs.	Lbs.	Lbs.
5 feet 3 inches	118	129	141
5 feet 4 inches	122	133	145
5 feet 5 inches	126	137	149
5 feet 6 inches	130	142	155
5 feet 7 inches	134	147	161
5 feet 8 inches	139	151	166
5 feet 9 inches	143	155	170
5 feet 10 inches	147	159	174
5 feet 11 inches	150	163	178
6 feet	154	167	183
6 feet 1 inch	158	171	188
6 feet 2 inches	162	175	192
6 feet 3 inches	165	178	195
Women			
5 feet	100	109	118
5 feet 1 inch	104	112	121
5 feet 2 inches	107	115	125
5 feet 3 inches	110	118	128
5 feet 4 inches	113	122	132
5 feet 5 inches	116	125	135
5 feet 6 inches	120	129	139
5 feet 7 inches	123	132	142
5 feet 8 inches	126	136	146
5 feet 9 inches	130	140	151
5 feet 10 inches	133	144	156
5 feet 11 inches	137	148	161
6 feet	141	152	166

(Adapted from U.S. Department of Agriculture Home and Garden Bulletin No. 74.)

Weight Control: The Computer Diet Method

able to choose among diet options. You will know numerically what will happen and when.) Finally, the computer diet is based on sound nutritional practices—no fads here. In short, you will be shown how to establish a *weight loss program* based on the following:

1. Set your weight loss goal and the rate at which you should lose weight.
2. Determine your Activity Level.
3. Determine your diet options from the Weight Loss Calorie Tables and choose the caloric intake and duration of your diet.
4. Analyze your eating habits and decide how you are going to spread your caloric intake—first among the days of the week, and then over the meals of an individual day.
5. Translate your caloric allowance into meal types and actual food portions by using the Weight Loss Diet Tables.

All of these points will be covered in much greater detail in subsequent chapters. You will be shown how to construct your own personalized weight loss program. Remember, dieting is not easy. However, be assured that if you stay with the program you develop, you will lose weight.

Computer Diet Weight Maintenance Program

Once the proper weight in relation to your height is achieved, your goal should be to maintain that weight level. As one of my professors used to remark constantly, "Easy to say, not so easy to do!" You may already know from experience that weight maintenance can be a very elusive goal indeed. Statistics show that more than ninety percent of all dieters regain every pound they have lost. It is easier to reduce than to stay reduced!

The subject of weight maintenance is usually ignored by most diet books. So the dieter who has somehow lost weight is left without any post-dieting guidelines to maintain his new weight level. Again, the computer diet maintenance program is different! For the first time you will be introduced to all the facts you need to understand in order to successfully maintain your lower weight. You will be shown how to apply the following to establish a *weight maintenance plan:*

1. Using the Weight Maintenance Calorie Tables, determine how many calories you may consume per day, without gaining or losing any significant amount of weight.
2. Analyze your eating habits and decide how you are going to spread your maintenance caloric allowance —first among the days of the week, and then over the meals of an individual day.
3. Translate caloric values into meal types and actual food portions by using the Weight Maintenance Menu Tables.

Again, each of these points will be elaborated on in subsequent chapters. But you must understand the components that comprise the total program before you can devise your own plan. So, for those readers who have prepared themselves mentally to start a weight control program, here is what you should know before you begin.

5. Weight Loss Calorie Tables

The first practical application of the weight control equations I described earlier resulted in the Weight Loss Calorie Tables. This series of tables, produced using a modern digital computer, represents the equivalent of 6000 man-hours of calculation. (If the calculations involved were done by hand, it would have taken four mathematicians, working full time, approximately one year to complete the task!) The tables make it possible to easily determine how long it will take to lose a desired amount of weight on a given reducing diet.

The Index on page 43 shows a summary of the Weight Loss Calorie Tables that follow. From the Index you can see that three height ranges are listed for males and two for females. Within each height range there are three age groups and for each age group, four page numbers are shown; these pages contain the Weight Loss Calorie Tables for a particular sex, height, and age group—for four different Activity Levels. All age groups have tables for Activity Levels 0 through 3, except for 18–35-year-old males, whose Activity Level range is 1 to 4.

How to Use the Weight Loss Calorie Tables

To use the Weight Loss Calorie Tables that follow, first determine your Activity Level as shown on page 14. Then find your personal Weight Loss Calorie Table—from

35

among the 60 tables included—by using the Index on page 43. At this point you are ready to use your table to determine specific diet options. This procedure is best explained by the following example: Consider a 32-year-old female, 5' 4" in height, weighing 140 pounds, whose physical activity is most closely described by Activity Level 2. From the Weight Loss Calorie Table Index, she finds that the Weight Loss Calorie Table which applies to her is contained on pages 80–83 (this group of pages is for Activity Levels 0 to 3). Then, by examining these pages, she finds that her personal table (for Activity Level 2) is on page 82. Assume that she wants to lose fifteen pounds. She uses the Weight Loss Calorie Table on page 82 as follows: First, she scans the far left edge of the table and locates a fifteen pound weight loss. She then sees four different diet options of 900, 1200, 1500, and 1800 calories. From this point, she proceeds horizontally to the right until she intersects the vertical column headed 140 pounds (her present weight); the four numbers in the intersected box correspond to her four diet options and represent the time in days that it will take her to lose fifteen pounds. Specifically, she determines that to lose fifteen pounds, her calorie intake options are:

1. 900 calories per day, for 40 days.
2. 1200 calories per day, for 50 days.
3. 1500 calories per day, for 68 days.
4. 1800 calories per day, for 106 days.

Actually, she has still another alternative: she could increase her daily energy expenditure at the same time. For example, assume that this woman decides to undertake a physical activity program that consists of a strenuous workout at home or in a gymnasium for more than one hour every day. In effect she has increased her Activity Level from 2 to 3 and finds on page 83 that now to lose fifteen pounds, her calorie intake options are:

1. 900 calories per day, for 32 days.
2. 1200 calories per day, for 39 days.
3. 1500 calories per day, for 49 days.
4. 1800 calories per day, for 66 days.

She may now decide which of the eight choices available is best for her. The selection process is a matter of deciding between relatively short-term low calorie diets and somewhat higher calorie but longer duration diets.

There is still another possibility, and that is not to reduce her caloric intake, but to increase only her physical activity. This, however, is not really a practical alternative except, perhaps, when a small amount of weight must be lost.

Interpolation

As a further illustration of the use of the Weight Loss Calorie Tables, suppose that the woman in the previous example weighed 150 pounds and wanted to lose fifteen pounds on a 1500 calorie diet. Now, 150 pounds is not listed on page 82. However, by noting that the length of time required to lose fifteen pounds at 150 pounds would be half-way between those at 140 and 160 pounds, she would proceed as follows. First, she would find that the length of time required at 140 pounds is 68 days and at 160 pounds, 54 days. The amount of time at 150 pounds would be in the middle of these two times, or 61 days. This estimating technique is called interpolation and should be used whenever you cannot find your exact weight in one of the tables.

If mathematics was never your strong suit, don't give up! Get a friend to help you. The important part—the doing—comes after the calculations. That's where you come in.

The Physiology of Weight Loss

The body weight lost during periods of negative energy balance is of variable composition. Fat, water, and protein are lost at different rates and at different times in the diet.

The amount of water in the human body also varies from day to day. Over a reasonable period of time, however, it can be stated that the amount of fluid leaving the body will equal the amount entering the body. The water balance of the body is then said to be in equilibrium.

A considerable loss of body water usually takes place at the start of a diet. Since one pint of water weighs approximately one pound, this initial water loss will appear to be a weight loss. But the weight loss is not "real," because no body tissue has been lost.* Many theories have been proposed to explain this phenomenon, but none have been confirmed scientifically. It is known that the water balance of the body is influenced by the amount of salt used in the diet, but research has shown that the initial high loss of water occurs even when adequate salt is used in the diet. So the reason for this phenomenon is still obscure.

Because of changes in body hydration, you will usually notice a higher weight loss during the first week or

---

* From this point on, when reference is made to "real" weight loss, what is meant is that weight loss which will not be regained, once the water balance of the body is restored.

two on a diet than the Weight Loss Calorie Tables predict. By the following week, however, the water balance of the body will again readjust and your total weight loss will more closely approach the values shown in the Weight Loss Calorie Tables. The tables are based on "real" weight loss. In addition, realize that the weight of a normal person will fluctuate two to three pounds daily. Your weight is lowest before breakfast and highest in the evening before retiring.

Another cause of weight fluctuation is water retention in women just prior to their menstrual period. This is not uncommon, and for the female dieter this may appear to be a time when weight is not lost. Again, the water balance of the body will reach equilibrium by the next week, when weight loss will once more closely follow the values shown in the Weight Loss Calorie Table.

After the period of high initial water loss, a difference of approximately 3500 calories between your food energy intake and your energy needs will result in a weight change of one pound.

Weight Loss Axioms

Once the parameters involved in weight loss are related in mathematical equation, it is possible, after studying the equations, to state some qualitative axioms. It is also possible to deduce the following principles, by examining the Weight Loss Calorie Tables.

1. Given two people on the same reducing diet, the heavier person will lose weight at the faster rate.
2. Given two people on the same reducing diet, the taller person will lose weight at the faster rate.
3. Given an individual on a reducing diet, if the caloric

intake is constant, the rate of weight loss will decrease as time increases. This is particularly evident in reducing diets of relatively long duration.
4. Given a male and female of the same age, weight, etc., on the same reducing diet, the male will lose weight faster than the female. In general, women need to eat less than men.
5. Given an individual whose caloric intake is constant over the years, this person will slowly gain weight, because the basal metabolic rate decreases as one advances in age.

Some of the axioms appear obvious; others are not so evident. In addition, by comparing Weight Loss Calorie Tables that differ in only one parameter—for example, sex, age, height, or Activity Level—the effect of that particular parameter on weight loss can be seen.

A Word of Caution

A reducing diet is best supervised by a physician. This is especially recommended when a great deal of weight needs to be lost, or when an individual has an ailment or a history of some medical problem. The Weight Loss Calorie Tables cover a wide range of values. And while the values in the tables are theoretically possible to attain, they are not necessarily recommended for everyone. The wide ranges shown were computed and included for the sake of completeness. Most physicians recommend that weight loss should be limited to two pounds per week, except for either very large individuals or if the total amount of weight to be lost is relatively small. In these cases an acceptable weight loss rate may be as high as three pounds per week.

Most nutritionists feel that reducing diets should not

have food intakes below 900 to 1200 calories. This is because it is difficult to obtain the proper amount of essential nutrients below these levels.

Fallacies Exposed

Another feature of the Weight Loss Calorie Tables is that they can be easily used to assess whether a weight loss claim is, or is not, possible. For example, a recent advertisement read, "Command your body to melt away fat . . . . Most women will lose five-six pounds the first week!"

Aside from the fact that most physicians do not recommend such a rapid weight loss, let's analyze the claim and see if it is even possible. First, I am going to interpret "most women" as most overweight women, and define said females as 5′ 4″, 140 pounds, 38 years old, and at Activity Level 1. Because the advertisement implies a long-term diet, I am going to assume that the caloric intake would not be less than 900. The rest is easy. From the Weight Loss Calorie Table on page 85, we find it will take the female just described 15 days to lose five pounds on a diet of 900 calories per day—or twice as long as the ad claimed!

As I have said before, the tables forecast how much "real" body weight will be lost. This woman's "real" weight loss in the first week would probably be more like two pounds, although a scale might show five pounds. The difference, of course, is due to the high initial loss of water which would eventually be equalized when fluid is retained, probably in the following week.

An interesting question related to this discussion would be: In theory, what is the fastest possible rate at which the woman in the preceding case could lose weight? That would naturally occur if she went on a total fast.

The calculation involved is beyond the scope of this book. But it can be shown that if the woman went on a true starvation diet (water only and not one calorie of food), it would take approximately nine days for her to lose five pounds of "real" weight. The advertisement not only promised a five pound weight loss in one week, but also guaranteed you would not be hungry!

Let me relate another example. I work out on Monday evenings at the YMCA. By 8 P.M., I have usually finished my last push-up and I am in the locker room. Invariably, a heavyweight will get on the scale and then shriek, "Damn it, I've gained five pounds over the weekend!" He walks away depressed and mutters, "One party and there goes my diet."

In this case, we don't need the Weight Loss Calorie Tables to analyze the situation—just common sense and some arithmetic. Recall what was said previously: ". . . a difference of approximately 3500 calories between your food energy intake and your energy needs will result in a weight change of one pound." Therefore, in order to gain five pounds over the weekend, the heavyweight would have had to eat 17,500 extra calories (3500 × 5) in two days! (This is in addition to his normal caloric intake for the two days.) I can state that it would be almost impossible to drink or eat the amount of food required for an excess of 17,500 calories in two days. How then can the five pound gain be explained? First, it is feasible that the man overate to the extent of a one or (at most) two pound "real" weight gain. The remainder of the weight gain is most likely due to a shift in his water balance.

In summary, when dieting you need patience. Don't be swayed by get-slim-quick schemes. There is no way to cheat nature—or the Weight Loss Calorie Tables, for that matter. Finally, be aware that changes in your body hydration can cause fluctuations in your weight which may not seem reasonable but which will be automatically corrected in time, as your water balance is restored.

WEIGHT LOSS CALORIE TABLE INDEX

SEX	HEIGHT	AGE	PAGE NOS.
MALE	5′ 0″—5′ 5″	18–35 36–55 56–75	44–47 48–51 52–55
MALE	5′ 6″—5′ 11″	18–35 36–55 56–75	56–59 60–63 64–67
MALE	6′ 0″—6′ 6″	18–35 36–55 56–75	68–71 72–75 76–79
FEMALE	4′ 11″—5′ 5″	18–35 36–55 56–75	80–83 84–87 88–91
FEMALE	5′ 6″—6′ 0″	18–35 36–55 56–75	92–95 96–99 100–103

WEIGHT LOSS CALORIE TABLE

Sex: Male Height 5' 0"—5' 5"
Age: 18–35 Yrs. Activity Level 1

WT. LOSS	DIET CALORIES	PRESENT WEIGHT LBS.							
		120	140	160	180	200	220	240	260
5	1200	20	17	14	12	11	10	9	8
5	1500	30	23	18	15	13	12	11	10
5	1800	58	36	26	21	17	15	13	11
5	2100		83	45	31	24	19	16	14
10	1200	43	35	29	26	23	20	19	17
10	1500	64	48	38	32	28	24	22	20
10	1800	129	76	55	43	36	30	27	24
10	2100		188	96	65	49	40	34	29
20	1200		73	61	53	47	42	39	36
20	1500		103	81	67	58	51	46	41
20	1800		172	119	92	75	64	56	49
20	2100			222	143	106	85	71	61
30	1200		116	97	83	73	66	60	55
30	1500		167	129	106	90	79	71	64
30	1800		301	195	147	118	100	87	77
30	2100				239	171	135	112	96
40	1200			135	115	101	90	82	75
40	1500			184	149	126	109	97	87
40	1800			291	211	167	139	120	106
40	2100				366	249	192	157	133
50	1200			178	150	131	116	105	96
50	1500			249	197	164	142	125	112
50	1800				287	222	183	156	136
50	2100					345	257	207	174
60	1200				189	163	144	129	118
60	1500				252	207	177	156	139
60	1800				383	286	231	195	170
60	2100						335	263	218
70	1200				232	198	174	155	141
70	1500				316	255	216	188	167
70	1800					363	286	239	206
70	2100							329	268

Values in table: time in days to lose weight indicated.

WEIGHT LOSS CALORIE TABLE

Sex: Male
Age: 18–35 Yrs.
Height: 5′ 0″—5′ 5″
Activity Level 2

WT. LOSS	DIET CALORIES	PRESENT WEIGHT LBS.							
		120	140	160	180	200	220	240	260
5	1200	17	14	12	10	9	8	8	7
5	1500	23	18	15	12	11	10	9	8
5	1800	37	25	19	16	13	11	10	9
5	2100	89	42	28	21	17	14	12	11
10	1200	35	29	25	21	19	17	16	14
10	1500	49	38	31	26	23	20	18	16
10	1800	80	53	40	33	28	24	21	19
10	2100	215	92	59	44	35	29	25	22
20	1200		61	52	45	40	36	33	30
20	1500		80	65	54	47	42	37	34
20	1800		118	87	69	58	50	44	39
20	2100		220	132	95	75	62	53	47
30	1200		97	81	70	62	55	50	46
30	1500		130	103	86	74	65	58	52
30	1800		198	141	110	91	78	68	61
30	2100			224	155	119	98	83	72
40	1200			113	97	85	76	69	63
40	1500			146	120	102	89	80	72
40	1800			205	157	128	108	94	84
40	2100			352	227	170	137	116	100
50	1200			149	126	110	98	88	81
50	1500			195	158	133	116	103	92
50	1800			285	210	168	141	122	108
50	2100				319	230	182	151	130
60	1200				159	137	121	109	99
60	1500				201	167	144	127	114
60	1800				275	215	178	153	134
60	2100					303	233	191	163
70	1200				194	167	146	131	119
70	1500				250	205	175	154	137
70	1800				355	269	219	186	162
70	2100					395	293	236	198

Values in table: time in days to lose weight indicated.

WEIGHT LOSS CALORIE TABLE

Sex: Male Height: 5′ 0″—5′ 5″
Age: 18–35 Yrs. Activity Level 3

WT. LOSS	DIET CALORIES	PRESENT WEIGHT LBS.							
		120	140	160	180	200	220	240	260
5	1200	13	11	9	8	7	7	6	5
5	1500	17	13	11	10	8	7	7	6
5	1800	23	17	14	11	10	8	8	7
5	2100	38	24	18	14	12	10	9	8
10	1200	28	23	20	17	15	14	13	11
10	1500	36	28	23	20	17	15	14	13
10	1800	50	36	29	24	20	18	16	14
10	2100	82	51	37	29	24	21	18	16
20	1200		49	41	36	32	29	26	24
20	1500		60	49	42	36	32	29	27
20	1800		79	61	50	43	37	33	30
20	2100		114	80	62	51	43	38	34
30	1200		77	65	56	49	44	40	37
30	1500		96	78	65	57	50	45	41
30	1800		129	98	79	67	58	51	46
30	2100		196	131	100	81	68	59	52
40	1200			90	77	68	61	55	51
40	1500			110	91	79	69	62	56
40	1800			140	111	93	80	71	63
40	2100			194	143	114	95	82	72
50	1200			119	101	88	79	71	65
50	1500			146	120	102	90	80	72
50	1800			190	148	122	104	91	81
50	2100			277	194	151	125	107	93
60	1200				127	110	97	88	80
60	1500				152	128	112	99	89
60	1800				191	155	131	114	101
60	2100				257	195	158	134	116
70	1200				155	133	117	105	95
70	1500				188	157	135	119	107
70	1800				241	191	160	138	121
70	2100				340	246	195	163	141

Values in table: time in days to lose weight indicated.

WEIGHT LOSS CALORIE TABLE

Sex: Male Height: 5' 0"—5' 5"
Age: 18–35 Yrs. Activity Level 4

WT. LOSS	DIET CALORIES	PRESENT WEIGHT LBS.							
		120	140	160	180	200	220	240	260
5	1200	9	8	7	6	5	5	4	4
5	1500	11	9	8	6	6	5	5	4
5	1800	14	11	9	7	6	6	5	4
5	2100	18	13	10	8	7	6	5	5
10	1200	20	16	14	12	11	10	9	8
10	1500	23	19	16	14	12	11	10	9
10	1800	29	22	18	15	13	12	11	10
10	2100	38	27	21	18	15	13	12	10
20	1200		35	30	26	23	21	19	17
20	1500		40	34	29	25	23	20	19
20	1800		48	39	33	28	25	22	20
20	2100		59	46	37	32	28	24	22
30	1200		55	46	40	36	32	29	27
30	1500		64	53	45	39	35	32	29
30	1800		77	62	51	44	39	35	31
30	2100		97	73	59	50	43	38	34
40	1200			65	56	49	44	40	37
40	1500			74	63	55	48	43	39
40	1800			87	72	61	53	48	43
40	2100			106	84	70	60	52	47
50	1200			85	73	64	57	51	47
50	1500			98	82	71	63	56	51
50	1800			117	95	80	69	61	55
50	2100			144	111	92	78	68	60
60	1200				91	79	71	63	58
60	1500				104	89	78	69	63
60	1800				120	100	87	76	68
60	2100				143	116	98	85	75
70	1200				111	96	85	76	69
70	1500				128	108	94	83	75
70	1800				150	123	105	92	82
70	2100				182	144	120	103	90

Values in table: time in days to lose weight indicated.

WEIGHT LOSS CALORIE TABLE

Sex: Male
Age: 36–55 Yrs.
Height: 5' 0"—5' 5"
Activity Level 0

WT. LOSS	DIET CALORIES	PRESENT WEIGHT LBS.							
		120	140	160	180	200	220	240	260
5	1200	25	20	17	15	13	12	11	10
5	1500	42	30	23	19	16	14	13	12
5	1800	123	56	37	28	22	19	16	14
5	2100			89	50	35	27	22	19
10	1200	52	42	35	30	27	24	22	20
10	1500	89	62	48	40	34	30	26	24
10	1800	300	122	78	58	46	39	33	29
10	2100			200	106	73	56	46	39
20	1200		89	74	63	56	50	45	41
20	1500		136	103	84	71	62	55	49
20	1800		294	173	125	98	82	70	61
20	2100				245	160	120	96	81
30	1200		142	116	99	86	77	70	64
30	1500		226	166	133	111	96	85	76
30	1800			296	203	157	128	109	95
30	2100					266	193	153	127
40	1200			163	137	119	106	95	87
40	1500			240	188	155	133	117	105
40	1800				299	224	180	152	132
40	2100						280	216	177
50	1200			216	179	155	136	123	111
50	1500			330	250	204	174	152	135
50	1800					302	239	199	171
50	2100						386	290	234
60	1200				226	193	169	151	137
60	1500				324	259	218	189	167
60	1800					398	306	251	214
60	2100							377	298
70	1200				279	236	205	182	164
70	1500					322	267	229	201
70	1800						384	309	261
70	2100								371

Values in table: time in days to lose weight indicated.

WEIGHT LOSS CALORIE TABLE

Sex: Male Height: 5' 0"—5' 5"
Age: 36–55 Yrs. Activity Level 1

WT. LOSS	DIET CALORIES	PRESENT WEIGHT LBS.							
		120	140	160	180	200	220	240	260
5	1200	23	18	15	13	12	11	10	9
5	1500	35	26	20	17	15	13	11	10
5	1800	80	44	30	23	19	16	14	12
5	2100		139	58	37	28	22	18	16
10	1200	47	38	32	27	24	22	20	18
10	1500	75	54	42	35	30	26	24	21
10	1800	182	93	64	49	40	34	29	26
10	2100		356	127	79	58	46	38	33
20	1200		80	67	57	51	45	41	38
20	1500		117	90	74	63	55	49	44
20	1800		217	140	104	84	70	61	54
20	2100			313	177	125	97	80	68
30	1200		128	105	90	79	70	63	58
30	1500		193	145	117	99	86	76	68
30	1800			234	169	133	111	95	83
30	2100				304	204	155	126	106
40	1200			147	125	108	96	87	79
40	1500			208	165	138	119	105	94
40	1800			357	245	189	155	132	115
40	2100					302	222	177	148
50	1200			195	163	141	124	112	102
50	1500			283	219	181	154	135	121
50	1800				339	253	204	172	149
50	2100						302	236	195
60	1200				205	176	154	138	125
60	1500				282	229	193	168	150
60	1800					329	260	216	186
60	2100							303	246
70	1200				253	214	187	166	150
70	1500				358	283	236	204	180
70	1800						324	265	226
70	2100							382	304

Values in table: time in days to lose weight indicated.

WEIGHT LOSS CALORIE TABLE

Sex: Male Height: 5' 0"—5' 5"
Age: 36–55 Yrs. Activity Level 2

WT. LOSS	DIET CALORIES	PRESENT WEIGHT LBS.							
		120	140	160	180	200	220	240	260
5	1200	18	15	13	11	10	9	8	7
5	1500	26	20	16	13	12	10	9	8
5	1800	45	29	22	17	14	12	11	10
5	2100	153	54	33	24	19	16	13	12
10	1200	38	31	26	23	20	18	17	15
10	1500	55	41	33	28	24	21	19	17
10	1800	98	61	45	36	30	26	23	20
10	2100		118	70	50	39	32	28	24
20	1200		66	55	48	42	38	34	31
20	1500		89	71	59	51	44	40	36
20	1800		137	98	76	63	54	47	42
20	2100		303	158	109	84	68	58	50
30	1200		105	87	75	65	58	53	48
30	1500		145	112	93	79	69	62	56
30	1800		235	159	122	99	84	73	65
30	2100			277	180	134	108	91	78
40	1200			122	103	90	80	73	66
40	1500			160	130	110	95	85	76
40	1800			235	174	140	117	101	90
40	2100				268	193	153	127	109
50	1200			161	135	117	104	93	85
50	1500			216	172	144	124	109	98
50	1800			333	236	186	154	132	116
50	2100				387	264	203	166	141
60	1200				170	146	129	115	105
60	1500				219	181	155	136	121
60	1800				312	238	194	165	144
60	2100					352	262	211	177
70	1200				209	178	155	139	125
70	1500				275	223	188	164	146
70	1800					300	240	201	174
70	2100						333	262	217

Values in table: time in days to lose weight indicated.

WEIGHT LOSS CALORIE TABLE

Sex: Male Height: 5' 0"—5' 5"
Age: 36–55 Yrs. Activity Level 3

WT. LOSS	DIET CALORIES	PRESENT WEIGHT LBS.							
		120	140	160	180	200	220	240	260
5	1200	14	12	10	9	8	7	6	6
5	1500	19	14	12	10	9	8	7	6
5	1800	26	19	15	12	10	9	8	7
5	2100	46	27	19	15	12	11	9	8
10	1200	30	24	21	18	16	14	13	12
10	1500	39	30	25	21	18	16	15	13
10	1800	56	40	31	25	22	19	17	15
10	2100	101	58	41	32	26	22	19	17
20	1200		52	43	38	33	30	27	25
20	1500		65	52	44	38	34	31	28
20	1800		87	66	54	45	39	35	31
20	2100		132	89	68	55	46	40	36
30	1200		82	68	59	52	46	42	38
30	1500		104	83	70	60	53	47	43
30	1800		144	106	85	71	61	54	48
30	2100		234	148	109	87	73	63	55
40	1200			96	82	72	64	58	53
40	1500			118	97	83	73	65	59
40	1800			153	120	99	85	74	66
40	2100			222	158	124	102	87	76
50	1200			126	106	93	82	74	67
50	1500			157	128	108	94	84	75
50	1800			210	161	131	111	97	86
50	2100			323	216	165	134	114	99
60	1200				134	115	102	91	83
60	1500				162	136	118	104	93
60	1800				208	166	139	120	106
60	2100				290	213	171	143	123
70	1200				164	140	123	110	100
70	1500				202	167	143	125	112
70	1800				264	206	171	146	128
70	2100				392	272	212	175	150

Values in table: time in days to lose weight indicated.

WEIGHT LOSS CALORIE TABLE

Sex: Male Height: 5' 0"—5' 5"
Age: 56–75 Yrs. Activity Level 0

WT. LOSS	DIET CALORIES	PRESENT WEIGHT LBS.							
		120	140	160	180	200	220	240	260
5	1200	29	23	19	16	14	13	11	10
5	1500	53	36	27	22	18	16	14	13
5	1800	329	81	47	34	26	22	18	16
5	2100			181	71	45	33	26	22
10	1200	60	47	39	33	29	26	24	22
10	1500	115	75	56	45	38	33	29	26
10	1800		181	100	70	54	44	38	33
10	2100				155	95	68	54	45
20	1200		101	82	70	61	54	49	45
20	1500		166	121	96	80	69	60	54
20	1800			229	153	116	94	79	69
20	2100				388	212	148	115	94
30	1200		162	130	109	95	84	75	69
30	1500		281	196	152	125	107	94	84
30	1800			254	187	149	124	107
30	2100					368	243	184	148
40	1200			183	152	131	115	103	94
40	1500			287	217	176	149	130	115
40	1800				383	269	210	174	148
40	2100						361	263	209
50	1200			244	200	170	149	133	120
50	1500				292	233	195	168	148
50	1800					370	281	228	193
50	2100							358	278
60	1200				253	213	185	165	149
60	1500				383	297	245	210	184
60	1800						364	290	243
60	2100								358
70	1200				314	261	225	198	178
70	1500					373	302	256	223
70	1800							361	298
70	2100								

Values in table: time in days to lose weight indicated.

WEIGHT LOSS CALORIE TABLE

Sex: Male Height: 5' 0"—5' 5"
Age: 56–75 Yrs. Activity Level 1

WT. LOSS	DIET CALORIES	PRESENT WEIGHT LBS.							
		120	140	160	180	200	220	240	260
5	1200	26	20	17	14	13	11	10	9
5	1500	43	30	23	19	16	14	12	11
5	1800	134	57	37	27	22	18	16	14
5	2100			88	48	34	26	21	18
10	1200	54	42	35	30	26	24	21	20
10	1500	92	63	48	39	33	29	26	23
10	1800	341	125	78	57	45	38	32	28
10	2100			199	103	70	54	44	37
20	1200		90	74	63	55	49	44	40
20	1500		138	103	83	70	61	54	48
20	1800		306	174	123	96	79	68	59
20	2100				240	155	115	92	77
30	1200		144	116	98	85	76	68	62
30	1500		231	167	132	110	94	83	74
30	1800			299	202	154	125	106	92
30	2100					258	186	146	121
40	1200			164	137	118	104	94	85
40	1500			242	187	154	131	115	102
40	1800				298	220	176	148	127
40	2100					395	270	208	170
50	1200			218	179	154	135	120	109
50	1500			335	251	202	171	148	132
50	1800				299	299	234	193	166
50	2100						374	279	224
60	1200				227	192	168	149	134
60	1500				326	258	215	185	163
60	1800					395	300	245	207
60	2100							363	286
70	1200				281	235	203	179	161
70	1500					321	264	225	197
70	1800						378	302	253
70	2100								356

Values in table: time in days to lose weight indicated.

WEIGHT LOSS CALORIE TABLE

Sex: Male Height: 5' 0"—5' 5"
Age: 56–75 Yrs. Activity Level 2

WT. LOSS	DIET CALORIES	PRESENT WEIGHT LBS.							
		120	140	160	180	200	220	240	260
5	1200	20	16	14	12	10	9	8	8
5	1500	30	22	18	15	13	11	10	9
5	1800	58	35	25	19	16	14	12	10
5	2100		76	41	28	21	17	15	13
10	1200	43	34	28	25	22	19	18	16
10	1500	64	47	37	31	26	23	20	18
10	1800	129	73	52	40	33	28	25	22
10	2100		174	87	59	45	36	30	26
20	1200		72	60	51	45	40	36	33
20	1500		101	78	64	55	48	43	38
20	1800		167	113	86	70	59	51	45
20	2100			204	130	96	77	64	55
30	1200		115	94	80	70	62	56	51
30	1500		166	125	102	86	75	66	59
30	1800		297	187	138	111	93	80	70
30	2100			378	218	156	122	101	86
40	1200			133	112	97	86	77	70
40	1500			180	143	120	103	91	81
40	1800			281	200	157	129	111	97
40	2100				334	227	174	141	120
50	1200			176	146	126	111	99	90
50	1500			244	190	157	134	118	105
50	1800				274	209	170	144	126
50	2100					315	233	187	156
60	1200				185	157	138	123	111
60	1500				245	199	168	146	130
60	1800				368	270	216	181	156
60	2100						304	238	197
70	1200				228	192	167	148	133
70	1500				309	246	205	177	157
70	1800					344	268	222	190
70	2100						392	298	242

Values in table: time in days to lose weight indicated.

WEIGHT LOSS CALORIE TABLE

Sex: Male   Height: 5' 0"—5' 5"
Age: 56–75 Yrs.   Activity Level 3

WT. LOSS	DIET CALORIES	PRESENT WEIGHT LBS.							
		120	140	160	180	200	220	240	260
5	1200	15	12	11	9	8	7	7	6
5	1500	21	16	13	11	9	8	7	7
5	1800	31	21	16	13	11	10	8	8
5	2100	59	32	22	17	14	11	10	9
10	1200	32	26	22	19	17	15	14	13
10	1500	43	33	27	23	19	17	15	14
10	1800	66	45	34	27	23	20	18	16
10	2100	136	69	46	35	28	24	21	18
20	1200		55	46	40	35	31	29	26
20	1500		71	57	47	41	36	32	29
20	1800		98	73	58	49	42	37	33
20	2100		160	102	76	60	50	43	38
30	1200		88	73	62	55	49	44	40
30	1500		115	90	75	64	56	50	45
30	1800		164	118	93	77	66	57	51
30	2100		296	171	123	96	79	68	59
40	1200			102	87	76	67	61	55
40	1500			128	105	89	77	69	62
40	1800			171	132	108	91	79	70
40	2100			263	178	136	111	94	82
50	1200			135	113	98	87	78	71
50	1500			172	138	116	100	89	80
50	1800			238	177	142	119	103	91
50	2100			399	247	183	147	123	106
60	1200				143	122	108	96	87
60	1500				176	146	125	110	98
60	1800				230	181	150	129	113
60	2100				339	239	187	155	132
70	1200				175	149	130	116	104
70	1500				220	179	152	133	118
70	1800				296	226	184	157	136
70	2100					308	234	191	161

Values in table: time in days to lose weight indicated.

WEIGHT LOSS CALORIE TABLE

Sex: Male Height: 5′ 6″—5′ 11″
Age: 18–35 Yrs. Activity Level 1

WT. LOSS	DIET CALORIES	PRESENT WEIGHT LBS.							
		140	160	180	200	220	240	260	280
10	1200	31	27	23	21	19	17	16	15
10	1500	42	34	29	25	22	20	18	17
10	1800	62	46	37	32	27	24	22	20
10	2100	120	73	53	42	35	30	26	23
20	1200		56	49	44	39	36	33	31
20	1500		72	61	53	47	42	38	35
20	1800		100	79	66	57	50	45	41
20	2100		164	115	89	74	63	55	49
30	1200		88	76	67	61	55	51	47
30	1500		114	95	82	72	65	59	54
30	1800		162	126	104	89	78	70	63
30	2100		285	189	143	116	98	85	75
40	1200			105	93	83	76	70	65
40	1500			133	114	100	89	81	74
40	1800			180	146	124	108	96	86
40	2100			280	205	164	137	118	104
50	1200			137	120	107	97	89	82
50	1500			175	148	129	115	104	95
50	1800			242	193	162	140	124	111
50	2100				279	217	179	153	134
60	1200				149	133	120	110	101
60	1500				186	161	142	128	116
60	1800				247	204	175	153	137
60	2100				370	279	227	192	167
70	1200				181	160	144	131	120
70	1500				228	195	171	153	139
70	1800				309	251	213	185	165
70	2100					353	280	234	202
80	1200					189	169	154	141
80	1500					233	203	181	163
80	1800					304	254	220	195
80	2100						342	282	241

Values in table: time in days to lose weight indicated.

WEIGHT LOSS CALORIE TABLE

Sex: Male Height: 5′ 6″—5′ 11″
Age: 18–35 Yrs. Activity Level 2

WT. LOSS	DIET CALORIES	PRESENT WEIGHT LBS.							
		140	160	180	200	220	240	260	280
10	1200	27	23	20	18	16	15	14	13
10	1500	34	28	24	21	19	17	15	14
10	1800	46	36	29	25	22	19	18	16
10	2100	72	50	38	31	27	23	20	18
20	1200		48	42	37	34	31	28	26
20	1500		59	50	44	39	35	32	29
20	1800		76	62	53	46	41	36	33
20	2100		109	82	66	56	48	43	38
30	1200		75	65	58	52	47	43	40
30	1500		93	78	68	60	54	49	45
30	1800		123	98	82	71	63	56	51
30	2100		181	132	105	87	75	66	59
40	1200			90	79	71	65	59	55
40	1500			109	94	83	74	67	62
40	1800			139	115	99	87	77	70
40	2100			191	149	122	104	91	81
50	1200			117	103	92	83	76	70
50	1500			143	122	107	95	86	79
50	1800			185	151	129	112	100	90
50	2100			264	199	161	136	118	105
60	1200				127	113	102	93	86
60	1500				153	133	118	106	97
60	1800				192	161	140	124	111
60	2100				258	205	171	147	130
70	1200				154	137	123	112	103
70	1500				187	161	142	128	116
70	1800				238	197	170	149	133
70	2100				330	255	210	179	157
80	1200					162	144	131	120
80	1500					192	168	150	136
80	1800					238	202	177	157
80	2100					314	254	214	186

Values in table: time in days to lose weight indicated.

WEIGHT LOSS CALORIE TABLE

Sex: Male Height: 5′ 6″—5′ 11″
Age: 18–35 Yrs. Activity Level 3

WT. LOSS	DIET CALORIES	PRESENT WEIGHT LBS.							
		140	160	180	200	220	240	260	280
10	1200	21	18	16	14	13	12	11	10
10	1500	26	22	19	16	15	13	12	11
10	1800	33	26	22	19	17	15	13	12
10	2100	44	33	27	22	19	17	15	14
20	1200		39	34	30	27	25	23	21
20	1500		46	39	34	30	28	25	23
20	1800		56	46	40	35	31	28	26
20	2100		71	56	47	40	35	32	28
30	1200		60	53	47	42	38	35	33
30	1500		72	61	53	47	43	39	36
30	1800		89	73	62	54	48	43	39
30	2100		115	90	74	63	55	49	44
40	1200			73	64	58	53	48	45
40	1500			85	74	65	59	53	49
40	1800			102	86	75	66	59	54
40	2100			128	104	88	76	67	60
50	1200			95	83	74	67	62	57
50	1500			111	96	84	75	68	63
50	1800			135	113	97	86	77	69
50	2100			172	137	115	99	87	78
60	1200				103	92	83	76	70
60	1500				120	105	93	84	77
60	1800				142	121	106	95	86
60	2100				175	145	123	108	96
70	1200				125	111	100	91	83
70	1500				146	127	112	101	92
70	1800				175	148	129	114	103
70	2100				220	178	150	131	116
80	1200					131	117	106	98
80	1500					151	133	119	108
80	1800					177	153	135	121
80	2100					216	180	155	137

Values in table: time in days to lose weight indicated.

WEIGHT LOSS CALORIE TABLE

Sex: Male Height: 5′ 6″—5′ 11″
Age: 18–35 Yrs. Activity Level 4

WT. LOSS	DIET CALORIES	PRESENT WEIGHT LBS.							
		140	160	180	200	220	240	260	280
10	1200	16	13	12	10	9	9	8	7
10	1500	18	15	13	11	10	9	9	8
10	1800	21	17	15	13	11	10	9	8
10	2100	25	20	17	14	12	11	10	9
20	1200		28	25	22	20	18	17	15
20	1500		32	27	24	22	20	18	17
20	1800		36	31	27	24	21	19	18
20	2100		43	35	30	26	23	21	19
30	1200		44	39	34	31	28	26	24
30	1500		50	43	38	34	30	28	26
30	1800		58	49	42	37	33	30	27
30	2100		68	56	47	41	36	33	30
40	1200			54	47	42	39	35	33
40	1500			60	52	46	42	38	35
40	1800			68	58	51	46	41	38
40	2100			78	66	57	50	45	41
50	1200			70	61	55	50	45	42
50	1500			78	68	60	54	49	45
50	1800			89	76	66	59	53	48
50	2100			104	86	74	65	58	52
60	1200				76	68	61	56	51
60	1500				85	74	66	60	55
60	1800				95	82	73	65	59
60	2100				109	92	81	71	64
70	1200				92	82	73	67	61
70	1500				103	90	80	72	66
70	1800				117	100	88	79	71
70	2100				134	113	98	86	77
80	1200					96	86	78	72
80	1500					107	94	85	77
80	1800					119	104	93	84
80	2100					136	116	102	91

Values in table: time in days to lose weight indicated.

WEIGHT LOSS CALORIE TABLE

Sex: Male Height: 5' 6"—5' 11"
Age: 36–55 Yrs. Activity Level 0

WT. LOSS	DIET CALORIES	PRESENT WEIGHT LBS.							
		140	160	180	200	220	240	260	280
10	1200	39	33	28	25	23	21	19	18
10	1500	56	44	37	32	28	25	23	21
10	1800	99	68	52	42	36	31	27	25
10	2100		143	87	63	50	41	35	31
20	1200		69	59	52	47	43	39	36
20	1500		94	77	66	58	52	47	43
20	1800		148	111	89	75	65	57	51
20	2100		360	195	136	105	86	74	64
30	1200		108	92	81	73	66	61	56
30	1500		150	122	103	90	80	72	66
30	1800		248	179	141	117	101	89	79
30	2100			339	224	169	137	115	100
40	1200			128	112	100	90	83	76
40	1500			172	144	124	110	99	90
40	1800			259	200	164	140	122	109
40	2100				332	242	192	161	138
50	1200			168	145	129	116	106	98
50	1500			228	188	161	142	127	115
50	1800			359	268	216	182	158	140
50	2100					330	256	211	180
60	1200				181	160	143	130	120
60	1500				238	202	176	157	142
60	1800				349	275	229	197	174
60	2100						329	267	225
70	1200				221	193	172	156	143
70	1500				294	247	213	189	170
70	1800					343	281	240	210
70	2100							330	275
80	1200					229	203	183	167
80	1500					296	254	223	200
80	1800						340	287	249
80	2100								331

Values in table: time in days to lose weight indicated.

WEIGHT LOSS CALORIE TABLE

Sex: Male Height: 5′ 6″—5′ 11″
Age: 36–55 Yrs. Activity Level 1

WT. LOSS	DIET CALORIES	PRESENT WEIGHT LBS.							
		140	160	180	200	220	240	260	280
10	1200	35	30	26	23	21	19	17	16
10	1500	49	39	33	28	25	22	20	19
10	1800	80	57	44	36	31	27	24	22
10	2100	212	102	68	51	41	35	30	27
20	1200		63	54	48	43	39	36	33
20	1500		83	69	59	52	46	42	38
20	1800		123	94	77	65	57	50	45
20	2100		239	149	110	88	73	63	55
30	1200		98	85	74	67	60	55	51
30	1500		132	108	92	81	72	65	59
30	1800		203	151	122	102	88	78	70
30	2100			252	178	139	115	98	86
40	1200			117	103	92	83	76	70
40	1500			152	128	111	99	89	81
40	1800			218	172	143	122	108	96
40	2100			389	260	198	161	136	119
50	1200			153	133	118	106	97	89
50	1500			202	168	145	128	114	104
50	1800			298	229	187	159	139	124
50	2100				362	266	213	178	154
60	1200				166	146	131	119	110
60	1500				212	181	158	141	128
60	1800				295	237	200	173	154
60	2100					348	272	224	192
70	1200				202	177	158	143	131
70	1500				261	220	192	170	153
70	1800				375	294	245	210	185
70	2100						340	276	234
80	1200	.				209	186	168	153
80	1500					264	228	201	180
80	1800					361	295	251	219
80	2100							335	280

Values in table: time in days to lose weight indicated.

WEIGHT LOSS CALORIE TABLE

Sex: Male Height: 5' 6"—5' 11"
Age: 36–55 Yrs. Activity Level 2

WT. LOSS	DIET CALORIES	PRESENT WEIGHT LBS.							
		140	160	180	200	220	240	260	280
10	1200	29	25	22	19	17	16	15	14
10	1500	38	31	26	23	20	18	17	15
10	1800	55	41	33	28	24	21	19	17
10	2100	97	61	45	36	30	26	23	20
20	1200		52	45	40	36	33	30	28
20	1500		66	55	48	42	38	34	32
20	1800		89	71	59	51	45	40	36
20	2100		137	98	77	63	54	47	42
30	1200		82	71	63	56	51	47	43
30	1500		105	87	75	66	59	53	49
30	1800		145	113	93	79	69	62	56
30	2100		234	160	123	100	85	74	65
40	1200			98	86	77	70	64	59
40	1500			122	104	91	81	73	67
40	1800			160	130	110	96	85	77
40	2100			236	175	141	118	102	90
50	1200			128	112	99	90	82	75
50	1500			161	135	118	104	94	85
50	1800			216	172	144	124	110	98
50	2100			333	237	187	155	133	116
60	1200				139	123	110	100	92
60	1500				170	147	129	116	105
60	1800				220	182	155	136	122
60	2100				313	239	195	166	145
70	1200				169	148	133	120	110
70	1500				209	178	156	139	126
70	1800				276	224	189	165	146
70	2100					301	241	203	175
80	1200					176	156	141	129
80	1500					213	185	164	148
80	1800					271	227	196	173
80	2100					377	294	243	209

Values in table: time in days to lose weight indicated.

WEIGHT LOSS CALORIE TABLE

Sex: Male Height: 5′ 6″—5′ 11″
Age: 36–55 Yrs. Activity Level 3

WT. LOSS	DIET CALORIES	PRESENT WEIGHT LBS.							
		140	160	180	200	220	240	260	280
10	1200	23	20	17	15	14	13	12	11
10	1500	29	24	20	18	16	14	13	12
10	1800	37	29	24	21	18	16	14	13
10	2100	52	38	30	25	21	18	16	15
20	1200		42	36	32	29	26	24	22
20	1500		50	42	37	33	29	27	25
20	1800		62	51	43	38	33	30	27
20	2100		82	64	52	44	38	34	31
30	1200		65	57	50	45	41	37	34
30	1500		79	66	57	51	46	41	38
30	1800		100	80	68	59	52	46	42
30	2100		135	102	82	69	60	53	47
40	1200			78	69	62	56	51	47
40	1500			93	80	70	63	57	52
40	1800			113	95	81	71	64	58
40	2100			146	116	97	83	73	65
50	1200			102	89	79	72	65	60
50	1500			122	104	91	81	73	66
50	1800			151	124	106	92	82	74
50	2100			199	154	127	108	95	84
60	1200				111	98	88	80	74
60	1500				130	113	100	90	82
60	1800				157	133	115	102	92
60	2100				199	161	136	118	104
70	1200				135	119	106	96	88
70	1500				159	137	121	108	98
70	1800				195	162	140	123	110
70	2100				252	199	166	143	126
80	1200					141	125	113	103
80	1500					163	143	127	115
80	1800					195	166	146	130
80	2100					243	200	170	149

Values in table: time in days to lose weight indicated.

WEIGHT LOSS CALORIE TABLE

Sex: Male Height: 5' 6"—5' 11"
Age: 56–75 Yrs. Activity Level 0

WT. LOSS	DIET CALORIES	PRESENT WEIGHT LBS.							
		140	160	180	200	220	240	260	280
10	1200	44	36	31	28	25	22	21	19
10	1500	66	51	42	35	31	27	25	22
10	1800	137	85	62	49	41	35	31	27
10	2100		250	119	79	60	48	40	35
20	1200		76	65	57	51	46	42	39
20	1500		109	88	74	64	57	51	46
20	1800		189	133	104	85	73	64	57
20	2100			280	175	128	102	85	73
30	1200		120	102	89	79	71	65	60
30	1500		175	139	116	100	88	79	71
30	1800		327	218	166	135	114	99	88
30	2100				294	208	162	133	114
40	1200			142	123	109	98	89	82
40	1500			197	162	138	121	108	98
40	1800			323	238	190	159	137	121
40	2100					304	231	187	158
50	1200			186	160	141	126	114	105
50	1500			264	213	180	157	139	126
50	1800				323	252	208	178	156
50	2100						310	247	207
60	1200				200	175	156	141	129
60	1500				271	226	196	173	155
60	1800					324	263	223	194
60	2100							316	261
70	1200				244	211	187	169	154
70	1500				338	278	238	208	186
70	1800						325	272	235
70	2100							396	321
80	1200					251	221	199	181
80	1500					336	284	247	219
80	1800						397	327	280
80	2100								389

Values in table: time in days to lose weight indicated.

WEIGHT LOSS CALORIE TABLE

Sex: Male Height: 5′ 6″—5′ 11″
Age: 56–75 Yrs. Activity Level 1

WT. LOSS	DIET CALORIES	PRESENT WEIGHT LBS.							
		140	160	180	200	220	240	260	280
10	1200	39	33	28	25	22	20	19	17
10	1500	57	44	37	31	27	24	22	20
10	1800	102	68	51	41	35	30	27	24
10	2100		145	86	62	48	40	34	30
20	1200		69	59	52	46	42	39	36
20	1500		95	77	65	57	51	46	42
20	1800		150	110	88	73	63	55	50
20	2100		372	194	134	103	84	71	62
30	1200		109	92	81	72	65	59	55
30	1500		152	122	102	89	78	70	64
30	1800		253	179	140	115	98	86	77
30	2100			340	220	165	132	111	96
40	1200			129	112	99	89	81	75
40	1500			172	143	123	108	97	88
40	1800			261	199	162	137	119	106
40	2100				329	237	187	155	133
50	1200			168	145	128	115	104	96
50	1500			229	188	160	140	124	112
50	1800			364	267	213	179	154	136
50	2100					323	249	204	173
60	1200				181	159	142	128	117
60	1500				238	200	174	154	139
60	1800				349	272	225	193	169
60	2100						321	258	217
70	1200				221	192	170	154	140
70	1500				295	245	211	186	166
70	1800					341	277	235	205
70	2100							320	266
80	1200					228	201	181	164
80	1500					295	251	220	196
80	1800						336	281	243
80	2100							393	321

Values in table: time in days to lose weight indicated.

WEIGHT LOSS CALORIE TABLE

Sex: Male Height: 5′ 6″—5′ 11″
Age: 56–75 Yrs. Activity Level 2

WT. LOSS	DIET CALORIES	PRESENT WEIGHT LBS.							
		140	160	180	200	220	240	260	280
10	1200	32	27	23	21	19	17	15	14
10	1500	43	34	29	25	22	20	18	16
10	1800	65	47	37	31	27	23	21	19
10	2100	133	75	53	41	34	29	25	22
20	1200		57	49	43	39	35	32	30
20	1500		73	61	52	46	41	37	34
20	1800		102	80	65	56	48	43	39
20	2100		172	116	88	71	60	52	46
30	1200		89	76	67	60	54	49	46
30	1500		117	96	81	71	63	57	52
30	1800		168	127	103	87	75	67	60
30	2100		305	191	141	113	94	81	71
40	1200			106	93	82	74	68	62
40	1500			134	113	98	87	78	71
40	1800			182	145	121	105	92	82
40	2100			288	204	159	131	112	98
50	1200			139	120	106	95	87	80
50	1500			178	148	127	112	100	91
50	1800			248	193	159	136	119	106
50	2100				280	213	173	146	127
60	1200				150	132	118	107	98
60	1500				187	159	139	124	112
60	1800				248	201	170	148	131
60	2100				376	275	220	184	159
70	1200				182	159	142	128	117
70	1500				230	194	168	149	134
70	1800				314	249	208	179	158
70	2100					351	273	225	193
80	1200					189	167	150	137
80	1500					233	200	176	158
80	1800					304	250	214	187
80	2100						336	272	230

Values in table: time in days to lose weight indicated.

WEIGHT LOSS CALORIE TABLE

Sex: Male Height: 5′ 6″—5′ 11″
Age: 56–75 Yrs. Activity Level 3

WT. LOSS	DIET CALORIES	PRESENT WEIGHT LBS.							
		140	160	180	200	220	240	260	280
10	1200	25	21	18	16	15	13	12	11
10	1500	31	25	22	19	17	15	14	12
10	1800	41	32	26	22	19	17	15	14
10	2100	61	43	33	27	23	20	17	16
20	1200		44	38	34	30	28	25	23
20	1500		54	45	39	35	31	28	26
20	1800		68	55	46	40	35	32	29
20	2100		93	70	57	48	41	36	33
30	1200		70	60	53	47	43	39	36
30	1500		85	71	61	54	48	44	40
30	1800		110	88	73	63	55	49	45
30	2100		155	114	90	75	64	57	50
40	1200			83	73	65	59	53	49
40	1500			100	85	74	66	60	55
40	1800			124	102	87	76	68	61
40	2100			164	128	105	90	78	69
50	1200			109	94	84	75	69	63
50	1500			131	111	96	85	77	70
50	1800			166	134	114	99	87	79
50	2100			226	171	138	117	101	90
60	1200				118	104	93	84	77
60	1500				139	120	106	95	86
60	1800				171	143	123	108	97
60	2100				222	176	147	126	111
70	1200				143	125	112	101	92
70	1500				171	146	128	114	103
70	1800				213	175	150	131	117
70	2100				283	219	180	154	134
80	1200					149	132	119	108
80	1500					175	152	135	121
80	1800					212	179	155	138
80	2100					270	218	184	159

Values in table: time in days to lose weight indicated.

WEIGHT LOSS CALORIE TABLE

Sex: Male Height: 6′ 0″—6′ 6″
Age: 18–35 Yrs. Activity Level 1

WT. LOSS	DIET CALORIES	PRESENT WEIGHT LBS.							
		160	180	200	220	240	260	280	300
10	1200	25	22	20	18	16	15	14	13
10	1500	31	27	23	21	19	17	16	15
10	1800	41	34	29	25	22	20	18	17
10	2100	61	46	37	31	27	24	22	20
20	1200		46	41	37	34	31	29	27
20	1500		56	49	43	39	36	33	31
20	1800		71	60	52	46	42	38	35
20	2100		99	79	66	57	50	45	41
30	1200		71	63	57	52	48	45	42
30	1500		87	76	67	61	55	51	47
30	1800		113	95	82	72	65	59	54
30	2100		161	126	104	89	78	69	63
40	1200			87	78	72	66	61	57
40	1500			105	93	83	76	70	64
40	1800			132	113	99	89	80	74
40	2100			179	146	123	108	96	86
50	1200			112	101	92	84	78	73
50	1500			137	120	107	97	89	82
50	1800			174	148	129	114	103	94
50	2100			240	192	161	139	123	111
60	1200				125	113	103	96	89
60	1500				149	132	120	109	101
60	1800				185	160	142	127	116
60	2100				245	203	174	153	137
70	1200				150	135	124	114	106
70	1500				180	160	144	131	120
70	1800				227	195	171	153	139
70	2100				307	250	212	185	164
80	1200					159	145	133	124
80	1500					189	169	153	141
80	1800					232	203	180	163
80	2100					303	254	219	194

Values in table: time in days to lose weight indicated.

WEIGHT LOSS CALORIE TABLE

Sex: Male Height: 6′ 0″—6′ 6″
Age: 18–35 Yrs. Activity Level 2

WT. LOSS	DIET CALORIES	PRESENT WEIGHT LBS.							
		160	180	200	220	240	260	280	300
10	1200	21	19	17	15	14	13	12	11
10	1500	26	22	20	18	16	15	13	12
10	1800	32	27	23	20	18	17	15	14
10	2100	44	34	29	24	21	19	17	16
20	1200		39	35	32	29	27	25	23
20	1500		47	41	36	33	30	28	26
20	1800		57	49	43	38	34	31	29
20	2100		74	60	51	45	40	36	33
30	1200		61	54	49	45	41	39	36
30	1500		73	64	57	51	47	43	40
30	1800		90	76	66	59	53	48	44
30	2100		118	95	80	70	62	55	50
40	1200			75	68	62	57	53	49
40	1500			88	78	70	64	59	54
40	1800			106	92	81	73	66	61
40	2100			134	112	96	85	76	69
50	1200			97	87	79	72	67	62
50	1500			114	101	90	82	75	69
50	1800			139	119	105	94	85	78
50	2100			179	147	126	110	98	89
60	1200				107	97	89	82	76
60	1500				125	111	101	92	85
60	1800				149	130	116	105	96
60	2100				186	157	137	121	109
70	1200				129	117	106	98	91
70	1500				151	134	121	110	101
70	1800				182	158	140	126	114
70	2100				230	192	166	146	131
80	1200					137	125	115	106
80	1500					158	142	129	118
80	1800					188	165	148	134
80	2100					231	197	173	154

Values in table: time in days to lose weight indicated.

WEIGHT LOSS CALORIE TABLE

Sex: Male Height: 6' 0"—6' 6"
Age: 18–35 Yrs. Activity Level 3

WT. LOSS	DIET CALORIES	PRESENT WEIGHT LBS.							
		160	180	200	220	240	260	280	300
10	1200	17	15	14	12	11	11	10	9
10	1500	20	18	16	14	13	12	11	10
10	1800	24	21	18	16	14	13	12	11
10	2100	30	25	21	18	16	14	13	12
20	1200		32	29	26	24	22	20	19
20	1500		37	33	29	26	24	22	21
20	1800		43	37	33	29	27	24	23
20	2100		52	44	38	33	30	27	25
30	1200		50	45	40	37	34	31	29
30	1500		58	51	45	41	37	34	32
30	1800		68	58	51	46	41	38	35
30	2100		83	69	59	52	46	42	38
40	1200			62	55	50	46	43	40
40	1500			70	62	56	51	47	43
40	1800			81	71	63	57	52	48
40	2100			97	82	72	64	58	52
50	1200			79	71	65	59	55	51
50	1500			91	80	72	65	60	56
50	1800			106	92	81	73	66	61
50	2100			127	107	93	82	74	67
60	1200				88	80	73	67	62
60	1500				100	89	81	74	68
60	1800				115	101	90	82	75
60	2100				135	116	102	91	83
70	1200				106	96	87	80	74
70	1500				120	107	97	88	81
70	1800				139	122	108	98	89
70	2100				166	141	123	110	99
80	1200					112	102	94	87
80	1500					126	114	103	95
80	1800					145	128	115	105
80	2100					169	147	130	117

Values in table: time in days to lose weight indicated.

WEIGHT LOSS CALORIE TABLE

Sex: Male Height: 6' 0"—6' 6"
Age: 18–35 Yrs. Activity Level 4

WT. LOSS	DIET CALORIES	PRESENT WEIGHT LBS.							
		160	180	200	220	240	260	280	300
10	1200	13	11	10	9	8	8	7	7
10	1500	14	13	11	10	9	8	8	7
10	1800	16	14	12	11	10	9	8	8
10	2100	19	16	14	12	11	10	9	8
20	1200		24	21	19	18	16	15	14
20	1500		26	23	21	19	17	16	15
20	1800		30	26	23	21	19	17	16
20	2100		34	29	25	22	20	18	17
30	1200		37	33	30	27	25	23	22
30	1500		41	36	33	29	27	25	23
30	1800		46	40	36	32	29	27	25
30	2100		53	45	39	35	31	29	26
40	1200			46	41	37	34	32	30
40	1500			50	45	40	37	34	31
40	1800			56	49	44	40	36	34
40	2100			63	54	48	43	39	36
50	1200			59	53	48	44	41	38
50	1500			65	58	52	47	43	40
50	1800			73	64	57	51	47	43
50	2100			82	71	62	56	50	46
60	1200				66	59	54	50	46
60	1500				72	64	58	53	49
60	1800				79	70	63	57	53
60	2100				88	77	69	62	57
70	1200					79	71	65	60	55
70	1500					87	77	70	64	59
70	1800					96	85	76	69	63
70	2100					108	94	83	75	68
80	1200						84	76	70	64
80	1500						91	82	75	69
80	1800						100	89	81	74
80	2100						111	98	88	80

Values in table: time in days to lose weight indicated.

WEIGHT LOSS CALORIE TABLE

Sex: Male Height: 6' 0"—6' 6"
Age: 36–55 Yrs. Activity Level 0

WT. LOSS	DIET CALORIES	PRESENT WEIGHT LBS.							
		160	180	200	220	240	260	280	300
10	1200	29	25	23	21	19	17	16	15
10	1500	38	32	28	25	22	20	19	17
10	1800	54	43	36	31	27	24	22	20
10	2100	93	64	50	41	35	30	27	24
20	1200		53	47	43	39	36	33	31
20	1500		67	58	51	46	42	39	36
20	1800		91	75	64	56	50	46	42
20	2100		141	106	86	72	63	55	50
30	1200		82	73	66	60	55	51	48
30	1500		105	90	80	71	65	59	55
30	1800		145	118	100	88	78	70	64
30	2100		234	171	136	113	98	86	77
40	1200			101	90	82	76	70	65
40	1500			125	110	98	89	81	75
40	1800			166	140	121	107	96	88
40	2100			247	192	159	136	119	106
50	1200			130	116	105	97	89	83
50	1500			164	142	126	114	104	96
50	1800			220	183	157	138	124	112
50	2100			340	257	209	177	154	136
60	1200				144	130	119	109	102
60	1500				177	156	140	128	117
60	1800				231	197	172	153	138
60	2100				334	265	222	191	169
70	1200				173	156	142	131	121
70	1500				215	189	169	153	140
70	1800				285	240	208	184	166
70	2100					330	272	233	204
80	1200					183	166	153	141
80	1500					224	199	179	164
80	1800					288	247	218	195
80	2100						328	278	242

Values in table: time in days to lose weight indicated.

WEIGHT LOSS CALORIE TABLE

Sex: Male Height: 6' 0"—6' 6"
Age: 36–55 Yrs. Activity Level 1

WT. LOSS	DIET CALORIES	PRESENT WEIGHT LBS.							
		160	180	200	220	240	260	280	300
10	1200	27	23	21	19	17	16	15	14
10	1500	34	29	25	22	20	18	17	16
10	1800	46	37	32	27	24	22	20	18
10	2100	73	53	42	35	30	26	23	21
20	1200		49	44	39	36	33	31	29
20	1500		61	53	47	42	38	35	33
20	1800		79	66	57	50	45	41	37
20	2100		115	89	74	63	55	49	44
30	1200		76	67	61	55	51	47	44
30	1500		95	82	72	65	59	54	50
30	1800		126	104	89	78	70	63	58
30	2100		189	143	116	98	85	75	68
40	1200			93	83	76	70	65	60
40	1500			114	100	89	81	74	68
40	1800			146	124	108	96	86	79
40	2100			205	164	137	118	104	93
50	1200			120	107	97	89	82	77
50	1500			148	129	115	104	95	87
50	1800			193	162	140	124	111	101
50	2100			279	217	179	153	134	120
60	1200				133	120	110	101	94
60	1500				161	142	128	116	107
60	1800				204	175	153	137	124
60	2100				279	227	192	167	148
70	1200				160	144	131	120	112
70	1500				195	171	153	139	128
70	1800				251	213	185	165	149
70	2100				353	280	234	202	179
80	1200					169	154	141	130
80	1500					203	181	163	149
80	1800					254	220	195	175
80	2100					342	282	241	211

Values in table: time in days to lose weight indicated.

WEIGHT LOSS CALORIE TABLE

Sex: Male Height: 6' 0"—6' 6"
Age: 36–55 Yrs. Activity Level 2

WT. LOSS	DIET CALORIES	PRESENT WEIGHT LBS.							
		160	180	200	220	240	260	280	300
10	1200	23	20	18	16	15	14	13	12
10	1500	28	24	21	19	17	15	14	13
10	1800	36	29	25	22	19	18	16	15
10	2100	50	38	31	27	23	20	18	17
20	1200		42	37	34	31	28	26	24
20	1500		50	44	39	35	32	29	27
20	1800		62	53	46	41	36	33	30
20	2100		82	66	56	48	43	38	35
30	1200		65	58	52	47	43	40	38
30	1500		78	68	60	54	49	45	42
30	1800		98	82	71	63	56	51	47
30	2100		132	105	87	75	66	59	54
40	1200			79	71	65	59	55	51
40	1500			94	83	74	67	62	57
40	1800			115	99	87	77	70	64
40	2100			149	122	104	91	81	73
50	1200			103	92	83	76	70	65
50	1500			122	107	95	86	79	73
50	1800			151	129	112	100	90	82
50	2100			199	161	136	118	105	94
60	1200				113	102	93	86	80
60	1500				133	118	106	97	89
60	1800				161	140	124	111	101
60	2100				205	171	147	130	116
70	1200				137	123	112	103	95
70	1500				161	142	128	116	107
70	1800				197	170	149	133	121
70	2100				255	210	179	157	140
80	1200					144	131	120	111
80	1500					168	150	136	125
80	1800					202	177	157	142
80	2100					254	214	186	165

Values in table: time in days to lose weight indicated.

WEIGHT LOSS CALORIE TABLE

Sex: Male   Height: 6' 0"—6' 6"
Age: 36–55 Yrs.   Activity Level 3

WT. LOSS	DIET CALORIES	PRESENT WEIGHT LBS.							
		160	180	200	220	240	260	280	300
10	1200	18	16	14	13	12	11	10	9
10	1500	22	19	16	15	13	12	11	10
10	1800	26	22	19	17	15	13	12	11
10	2100	33	27	22	19	17	15	14	12
20	1200		34	30	27	25	23	21	20
20	1500		39	34	30	28	25	23	21
20	1800		46	40	35	31	28	26	24
20	2100		56	47	40	35	32	28	26
30	1200		53	47	42	38	35	33	30
30	1500		61	53	47	43	39	36	33
30	1800		73	62	54	48	43	39	36
30	2100		90	74	63	55	49	44	40
40	1200			64	58	53	48	45	41
40	1500			74	65	59	53	49	45
40	1800			86	75	66	59	54	50
40	2100			104	88	76	67	60	55
50	1200			83	74	67	62	57	53
50	1500			96	84	75	68	63	58
50	1800			113	97	86	77	69	64
50	2100			137	115	99	87	78	71
60	1200				92	83	76	70	65
60	1500				105	93	84	77	71
60	1800				121	106	95	86	78
60	2100				145	123	108	96	87
70	1200				111	100	91	83	77
70	1500				127	112	101	92	85
70	1800				148	129	114	103	93
70	2100				178	150	131	116	104
80	1200					117	106	98	90
80	1500					133	119	108	99
80	1800					153	135	121	110
80	2100					180	155	137	123

Values in table: time in days to lose weight indicated.

WEIGHT LOSS CALORIE TABLE

Sex: Male　　　Height: 6' 0"—6' 6"
Age: 56–75 Yrs.　Activity Level 0

WT. LOSS	DIET CALORIES	PRESENT WEIGHT LBS.							
		160	180	200	220	240	260	280	300
10	1200	32	28	25	22	20	19	17	16
10	1500	43	36	31	27	24	22	20	19
10	1800	65	50	41	35	30	27	24	22
10	2100	132	82	60	48	40	34	30	27
20	1200		58	51	46	42	39	36	34
20	1500		75	65	57	51	46	42	39
20	1800		107	86	73	63	56	50	46
20	2100		184	130	102	84	72	63	56
30	1200		91	80	72	65	60	55	51
30	1500		119	101	88	78	71	65	59
30	1800		172	137	114	98	87	78	70
30	2100		316	213	163	132	112	97	86
40	1200			110	98	89	81	75	70
40	1500			140	122	108	97	88	81
40	1800			194	160	136	119	107	96
40	2100			315	233	186	156	135	119
50	1200			143	127	114	104	96	89
50	1500			184	158	139	125	113	104
50	1800			259	210	178	155	137	124
50	2100				315	247	204	175	153
60	1200				157	141	128	118	109
60	1500				197	173	154	139	127
60	1800				267	223	193	170	153
60	2100					317	258	219	191
70	1200				189	169	153	141	130
70	1500				241	209	185	167	152
70	1800				332	274	234	205	184
70	2100						319	267	231
80	1200					200	180	165	152
80	1500					249	219	196	178
80	1800					331	280	243	216
80	2100						389	321	275

Values in table: time in days to lose weight indicated.

WEIGHT LOSS CALORIE TABLE

Sex: Male Height: 6' 0"—6' 6"
Age: 56–75 Yrs. Activity Level 1

WT. LOSS	DIET CALORIES	PRESENT WEIGHT LBS.							
		160	180	200	220	240	260	280	300
10	1200	29	26	23	20	19	17	16	15
10	1500	38	32	28	24	22	20	18	17
10	1800	55	43	36	30	27	24	21	20
10	2100	96	65	49	40	34	29	26	23
20	1200		53	47	42	39	36	33	31
20	1500		67	58	51	46	41	38	35
20	1800		92	75	64	56	49	45	41
20	2100		143	106	85	71	61	54	48
30	1200		83	73	66	60	55	51	47
30	1500		106	90	79	71	64	58	54
30	1800		147	118	100	87	77	69	63
30	2100		239	171	135	112	96	84	75
40	1200			101	90	82	75	69	64
40	1500			126	109	97	87	80	73
40	1800			167	139	120	106	95	86
40	2100			249	192	157	133	116	103
50	1200			131	116	105	96	88	82
50	1500			164	142	125	112	102	94
50	1800			222	183	156	136	122	110
50	2100			345	257	207	174	150	133
60	1200				144	129	118	108	100
60	1500				177	156	139	126	115
60	1800				231	195	170	151	136
60	2100				335	263	218	188	165
70	1200				174	155	141	129	119
70	1500				216	188	167	151	138
70	1800				286	239	206	182	163
70	2100					329	268	228	199
80	1200					183	165	151	139
80	1500					223	197	177	161
80	1800					287	245	215	192
80	2100						325	273	236

Values in table: time in days to lose weight indicated.

WEIGHT LOSS CALORIE TABLE

Sex: Male Height: 6' 0"—6' 6"
Age: 56–75 Yrs. Activity Level 2

WT. LOSS	DIET CALORIES	PRESENT WEIGHT LBS.							
		160	180	200	220	240	260	280	300
10	1200	25	21	19	17	16	14	13	12
10	1500	31	26	23	20	18	16	15	14
10	1800	40	33	28	24	21	19	17	16
10	2100	59	44	35	29	25	22	20	18
20	1200		45	40	36	33	30	28	26
20	1500		54	47	42	37	34	31	29
20	1800		69	58	50	44	39	36	33
20	2100		95	75	62	53	47	41	37
30	1200		70	62	55	50	46	43	40
30	1500		86	74	65	58	52	48	44
30	1800		110	91	78	68	61	55	50
30	2100		155	119	98	83	72	64	58
40	1200			85	76	69	63	58	54
40	1500			102	89	80	72	66	61
40	1800			128	108	94	84	75	69
40	2100			170	137	116	100	88	79
50	1200			110	98	88	81	74	69
50	1500			133	116	103	92	84	77
50	1800			168	141	122	108	97	88
50	2100			230	182	151	130	114	102
60	1200				121	109	99	91	85
60	1500				144	127	114	104	95
60	1800				178	153	134	120	108
60	2100				233	191	163	142	126
70	1200				146	131	119	109	101
70	1500				175	154	137	124	114
70	1800				219	186	162	144	130
70	2100				293	236	198	172	152
80	1200					154	140	128	118
80	1500					182	162	146	133
80	1800					222	192	170	153
80	2100					287	238	205	180

Values in table: time in days to lose weight indicated.

WEIGHT LOSS CALORIE TABLE

Sex: Male Height: 6' 0"—6' 6"
Age: 56–75 Yrs. Activity Level 3

WT. LOSS	DIET CALORIES	PRESENT WEIGHT LBS.							
		160	180	200	220	240	260	280	300
10	1200	20	17	15	14	13	11	11	10
10	1500	23	20	17	15	14	13	12	11
10	1800	29	24	20	18	16	14	13	12
10	2100	37	29	24	21	18	16	15	13
20	1200		36	32	29	26	24	22	21
20	1500		42	36	32	29	27	24	23
20	1800		50	43	37	33	30	27	25
20	2100		62	51	43	38	34	30	28
30	1200		56	49	44	40	37	34	32
30	1500		65	57	50	45	41	38	35
30	1800		79	67	58	51	46	42	38
30	2100		100	81	68	59	52	47	43
40	1200			68	61	55	51	47	43
40	1500			79	69	62	56	51	47
40	1800			93	80	71	63	57	52
40	2100			114	95	82	72	64	58
50	1200			88	79	71	65	60	55
50	1500			102	90	80	72	66	61
50	1800			122	104	91	81	73	67
50	2100			151	125	107	93	83	75
60	1200				97	88	80	73	68
60	1500				112	99	89	81	74
60	1800				131	114	101	91	82
60	2100				158	134	116	103	92
70	1200				117	105	95	87	81
70	1500				135	119	107	97	89
70	1800				160	138	121	109	99
70	2100				195	163	141	124	111
80	1200					124	112	102	94
80	1500					141	126	114	104
80	1800					164	144	128	116
80	2100					196	168	147	131

Values in table: time in days to lose weight indicated.

WEIGHT LOSS CALORIE TABLE

Sex: Female Height: 4' 11"—5' 5"
Age: 18–35 Yrs. Activity Level 0

WT. LOSS	DIET CALORIES	PRESENT WEIGHT LBS.							
		110	120	130	140	160	180	200	220
5	900	21	19	17	16	14	12	11	10
5	1200	31	27	24	21	18	15	13	12
5	1500	61	47	38	32	25	20	17	15
5	1800		175	95	66	41	30	24	20
10	900	43	39	35	33	28	25	23	21
10	1200	65	56	49	44	37	32	28	25
10	1500	133	100	81	68	52	42	36	31
10	1800			219	144	87	63	50	41
15	900		60	55	50	44	39	35	32
15	1200		87	77	68	57	49	43	38
15	1500		161	128	106	80	65	55	48
15	1800			394	240	138	99	77	64
20	900		82	75	69	59	52	47	43
20	1200		122	106	94	77	66	58	52
20	1500		233	181	149	111	89	75	65
20	1800				364	196	137	106	87
30	900			118	108	93	81	73	66
30	1200			171	151	122	103	90	80
30	1500			314	249	179	141	118	101
30	1800					341	225	170	137
40	900				152	129	112	100	91
40	1200				216	172	144	125	110
40	1500				383	260	201	165	140
40	1800						334	243	194
50	900					168	146	129	116
50	1200					228	189	162	142
50	1500					361	269	217	183
50	1800							331	257
60	900					211	182	160	144
60	1200					294	238	202	177
60	1500						350	276	230
60	1800								331

Values in table: time in days to lose weight indicated.

WEIGHT LOSS CALORIE TABLE

Sex: Female   Height: 4' 11"—5' 5"
Age: 18–35 Yrs.   Activity Level 1

WT. LOSS	DIET CALORIES	PRESENT WEIGHT LBS.							
		110	120	130	140	160	180	200	220
5	900	19	17	16	15	13	11	10	9
5	1200	28	24	21	19	16	14	12	11
5	1500	49	39	32	28	22	18	15	13
5	1800	210	99	66	49	33	25	20	17
10	900	40	36	33	30	26	23	21	19
10	1200	58	50	44	40	33	29	25	23
10	1500	106	82	68	58	45	37	32	28
10	1800		234	145	106	70	52	42	35
15	900		55	51	46	40	36	32	29
15	1200		78	69	62	51	44	39	35
15	1500		132	107	91	70	57	49	42
15	1800			245	172	110	81	65	55
20	900		76	69	63	55	48	44	40
20	1200		108	95	85	70	60	53	47
20	1500		188	151	126	96	78	66	58
20	1800			380	252	154	113	89	74
30	900			109	100	86	75	67	61
30	1200			153	135	110	94	82	73
30	1500			257	209	155	124	104	90
30	1800					261	183	142	117
40	900				140	119	104	92	84
40	1200				193	155	130	113	100
40	1500				315	223	175	145	124
40	1800						267	203	164
50	900				185	155	134	119	107
50	1200				262	205	170	147	129
50	1500					306	233	190	162
50	1800						374	273	217
60	900				237	195	168	148	133
60	1200				348	264	215	183	160
60	1500						302	242	203
60	1800							357	277

Values in table: time in days to lose weight indicated.

WEIGHT LOSS CALORIE TABLE

Sex: Female Height: 4′ 11″—5′ 5″
Age: 18–35 Yrs. Activity Level 2

WT. LOSS	DIET CALORIES	PRESENT WEIGHT LBS.							
		110	120	130	140	160	180	200	220
5	900	16	15	13	12	11	10	9	8
5	1200	22	19	17	16	13	11	10	9
5	1500	34	28	24	21	17	14	12	11
5	1800	73	50	39	31	23	18	15	13
10	900	34	31	28	26	22	20	18	16
10	1200	46	40	36	32	27	24	21	19
10	1500	72	59	50	44	35	29	25	22
10	1800	168	110	83	67	48	38	31	27
15	900		47	43	40	34	30	27	25
15	1200		63	56	50	42	36	32	29
15	1500		94	79	68	54	45	39	34
15	1800		184	134	106	75	59	48	41
20	900		65	59	54	47	41	37	34
20	1200		87	77	69	57	49	43	39
20	1500		132	110	94	74	61	53	46
20	1800		279	194	150	104	81	66	56
30	900			93	85	73	64	57	52
30	1200			123	110	90	77	68	60
30	1500			183	154	118	97	82	72
30	1800			362	261	172	129	105	88
40	900				120	102	89	79	71
40	1200				156	127	107	93	83
40	1500				227	169	136	114	99
40	1800					255	186	147	123
50	900				158	133	115	102	92
50	1200				211	168	140	121	107
50	1500				321	229	180	150	129
50	1800					366	253	196	161
60	900				202	167	143	126	113
60	1200				277	214	177	151	133
60	1500					302	231	189	161
60	1800						336	252	204

Values in table: time in days to lose weight indicated.

WEIGHT LOSS CALORIE TABLE

Sex: Female Height: 4' 11"—5' 5"
Age: 18–35 Yrs. Activity Level 3

WT. LOSS	DIET CALORIES	PRESENT WEIGHT LBS.							
		110	120	130	140	160	180	200	220
5	900	13	12	11	10	9	8	7	6
5	1200	17	15	13	12	10	9	8	7
5	1500	23	19	17	15	12	10	9	8
5	1800	36	28	23	20	15	13	11	9
10	900	27	25	23	21	18	16	14	13
10	1200	35	31	28	25	21	18	16	15
10	1500	48	41	36	31	26	22	19	17
10	1800	78	60	49	42	32	26	22	19
15	900		38	35	32	28	25	22	20
15	1200		48	43	39	33	28	25	23
15	1500		64	55	49	40	33	29	26
15	1800		97	78	66	50	41	34	30
20	900		53	48	44	38	34	30	27
20	1200		66	59	53	45	39	34	31
20	1500		90	77	67	54	46	40	35
20	1800		139	110	92	69	56	47	41
30	900			76	69	59	52	47	42
30	1200			95	85	70	60	53	48
30	1500			126	109	86	72	62	54
30	1800			189	153	112	89	74	63
40	900				97	83	72	64	58
40	1200				120	99	84	73	65
40	1500				158	122	101	86	75
40	1800				231	162	125	103	88
50	900				128	108	93	83	74
50	1200				161	130	110	95	84
50	1500				218	164	133	112	97
50	1800				343	222	168	136	115
60	900				164	136	117	103	92
60	1200				210	165	138	119	105
60	1500				295	213	169	141	121
60	1800					301	218	173	144

Values in table: time in days to lose weight indicated.

WEIGHT LOSS CALORIE TABLE

Sex: Female Height: 4' 11"—5' 5"
Age: 36–55 Yrs. Activity Level 0

WT. LOSS	DIET CALORIES	PRESENT WEIGHT LBS.							
		110	120	130	140	160	180	200	220
5	900	22	20	18	17	14	13	11	10
5	1200	34	29	25	23	19	16	14	13
5	1500	72	53	43	36	27	22	18	16
5	1800		329	129	81	47	34	26	22
10	900	46	41	37	34	30	26	24	22
10	1200	71	60	53	47	39	33	29	26
10	1500	159	115	90	75	56	45	38	33
10	1800			313	181	100	70	54	44
15	900		63	58	53	46	40	36	33
15	1200		95	82	73	60	51	45	40
15	1500		187	144	118	87	70	58	50
15	1800				310	160	110	84	69
20	900		87	79	72	62	55	49	45
20	1200		132	114	101	82	70	61	54
20	1500		275	206	166	121	96	80	69
20	1800					229	153	116	94
30	900			125	114	97	85	76	69
30	1200			185	162	130	109	95	84
30	1500			366	281	196	152	125	107
30	1800						254	187	149
40	900				160	135	117	104	94
40	1200				233	183	152	131	115
40	1500					287	217	176	149
40	1800						383	269	210
50	900				212	176	152	134	121
50	1200				320	244	200	170	149
50	1500						292	233	195
50	1800							370	281
60	900				271	222	190	167	149
60	1200					315	253	213	185
60	1500						383	297	245
60	1800								364

Values in table: time in days to lose weight indicated.

WEIGHT LOSS CALORIE TABLE

Sex: Female　　Height: 4' 11"—5' 5"
Age: 36–55 Yrs.　Activity Level 1

WT. LOSS	DIET CALORIES	PRESENT WEIGHT LBS.							
		110	120	130	140	160	180	200	220
5	900	20	18	17	15	13	12	10	10
5	1200	30	26	23	20	17	14	13	11
5	1500	56	43	35	30	23	19	16	14
5	1800		134	80	57	37	27	22	18
10	900	42	38	34	32	27	24	22	20
10	1200	62	54	47	42	35	30	26	24
10	1500	122	92	75	63	48	39	33	29
10	1800		341	181	125	78	57	45	38
15	900		58	53	49	42	37	33	30
15	1200		84	73	65	54	46	40	36
15	1500		149	118	99	75	61	51	45
15	1800			316	205	123	89	70	58
20	900		80	72	66	57	50	45	41
20	1200		116	101	90	74	63	55	49
20	1500		215	168	138	103	83	70	61
20	1800				306	174	123	96	79
30	900			115	105	89	78	70	63
30	1200			164	144	116	98	85	76
30	1500			290	231	167	132	110	94
30	1800					299	202	154	125
40	900				147	124	108	96	87
40	1200				207	164	137	118	104
40	1500				353	242	187	154	131
40	1800						298	220	176
50	900				194	162	140	124	111
50	1200				282	218	179	154	135
50	1500					335	251	202	171
50	1800							299	234
60	900				249	204	175	154	137
60	1200				377	281	227	192	168
60	1500						326	258	215
60	1800							395	300

Values in table: time in days to lose weight indicated.

WEIGHT LOSS CALORIE TABLE

Sex: Female Height: 4' 11"—5' 5"
Age: 36–55 Yrs. Activity Level 2

WT. LOSS	DIET CALORIES	PRESENT WEIGHT LBS.							
		110	120	130	140	160	180	200	220
5	900	17	15	14	13	11	10	9	8
5	1200	23	20	18	16	14	12	10	9
5	1500	37	30	26	22	18	15	13	11
5	1800	90	58	43	35	25	19	16	14
10	900	35	32	29	27	23	20	18	17
10	1200	49	43	38	34	28	25	22	19
10	1500	80	64	54	47	37	31	26	23
10	1800	214	129	93	73	52	40	33	28
15	900		49	45	41	36	31	28	26
15	1200		66	59	53	44	38	33	30
15	1500		102	85	73	57	47	40	35
15	1800		219	152	117	81	62	51	43
20	900		68	61	56	48	43	38	35
20	1200		92	81	72	60	51	45	40
20	1500		144	119	101	78	64	55	48
20	1800		344	223	167	113	86	70	59
30	900			97	89	76	66	59	54
30	1200			130	115	94	80	70	62
30	1500			199	166	125	102	86	75
30	1800				297	187	138	111	93
40	900				124	105	92	81	74
40	1200				165	133	112	97	86
40	1500				246	180	143	120	103
40	1800					281	200	157	129
50	900				165	138	119	105	94
50	1200				223	176	146	126	111
50	1500				352	244	190	157	134
50	1800						274	209	170
60	900				211	173	149	130	117
60	1200				295	225	185	157	138
60	1500					325	245	199	168
60	1800						368	270	216

Values in table: time in days to lose weight indicated.

WEIGHT LOSS CALORIE TABLE

Sex: Female Height: 4′ 11″—5′ 5″
Age: 36–55 Yrs. Activity Level 3

WT. LOSS	DIET CALORIES	PRESENT WEIGHT LBS.							
		110	120	130	140	160	180	200	220
5	900	14	12	11	10	9	8	7	6
5	1200	17	15	14	12	11	9	8	7
5	1500	24	21	18	16	13	11	9	8
5	1800	40	31	25	21	16	13	11	10
10	900	28	26	23	22	19	16	15	13
10	1200	37	32	29	26	22	19	17	15
10	1500	52	43	37	33	27	23	19	17
10	1800	87	66	53	45	34	27	23	20
15	900		40	36	33	29	25	23	21
15	1200		50	45	40	34	29	26	23
15	1500		68	58	51	41	35	30	26
15	1800		106	84	70	53	42	36	31
20	900		54	49	45	39	34	31	28
20	1200		69	61	55	46	40	35	31
20	1500		95	81	71	57	47	41	36
20	1800		153	119	98	73	58	49	42
30	900			78	72	61	54	48	43
30	1200			99	88	73	62	55	49
30	1500			133	115	90	75	64	56
30	1800			206	164	118	93	77	66
40	900				100	85	74	66	59
40	1200				125	102	87	76	67
40	1500				167	128	105	89	77
40	1800				251	171	132	108	91
50	900				133	111	96	85	76
50	1200				168	135	113	98	87
50	1500				231	172	138	116	100
50	1800				381	238	177	142	119
60	900				169	140	120	105	94
60	1200				220	172	143	122	108
60	1500				316	224	176	146	125
60	1800					325	230	181	150

Values in table: time in days to lose weight indicated.

WEIGHT LOSS CALORIE TABLE

Sex: Female Height: 4′ 11″—5′ 5″
Age: 56–75 Yrs. Activity Level 0

WT. LOSS	DIET CALORIES	PRESENT WEIGHT LBS.							
		110	120	130	140	160	180	200	220
5	900	24	22	20	18	15	14	12	11
5	1200	39	33	29	25	21	18	15	14
5	1500	101	69	52	42	31	25	20	18
5	1800			292	127	61	40	30	24
10	900	50	45	41	37	32	28	25	23
10	1200	83	69	60	53	43	36	32	28
10	1500	234	151	112	90	65	51	42	36
10	1800				304	131	85	63	51
15	900		69	63	57	49	43	39	35
15	1200		109	93	82	66	56	48	43
15	1500		252	181	143	101	79	65	55
15	1800					213	134	98	78
20	900		95	86	78	67	59	52	47
20	1200		152	129	113	91	76	66	58
20	1500		385	263	202	140	108	89	76
20	1800					313	188	136	107
30	900			136	124	105	91	81	73
30	1200			212	182	144	119	103	90
30	1500				354	230	174	140	118
30	1800						319	221	171
40	900				174	146	126	111	100
40	1200				266	204	167	143	125
40	1500					343	249	198	165
40	1800							325	244
50	900				232	191	164	144	129
50	1200				369	274	220	186	162
50	1500						339	263	216
50	1800								329
60	900				299	242	205	179	159
60	1200					357	281	234	201
60	1500							338	274
60	1800								

Values in table: time in days to lose weight indicated.

WEIGHT LOSS CALORIE TABLE

Sex: Female Height: 4' 11"—5' 5"
Age: 56–75 Yrs. Activity Level 1

WT. LOSS	DIET CALORIES	PRESENT WEIGHT LBS.							
		110	120	130	140	160	180	200	220
5	900	22	20	18	16	14	12	11	10
5	1200	34	29	25	22	18	16	14	12
5	1500	72	53	42	35	26	21	18	15
5	1800	0	311	122	77	45	32	25	20
10	900	46	41	37	34	29	26	23	21
10	1200	71	60	52	46	38	32	28	25
10	1500	161	114	89	73	55	44	37	32
10	1800			297	172	95	67	51	42
15	900		63	57	52	45	39	35	32
15	1200		94	82	72	59	50	43	39
15	1500		187	142	116	85	67	56	48
15	1800				295	152	104	80	65
20	900		87	78	72	61	54	48	43
20	1200		132	113	99	80	68	59	52
20	1500		275	204	163	117	93	77	66
20	1800					218	145	110	89
30	900			125	113	96	83	74	67
30	1200			185	160	127	107	92	81
30	1500			365	277	191	148	121	103
30	1800					390	241	177	141
40	900				159	133	115	102	92
40	1200				232	180	149	128	112
40	1500					281	211	170	143
40	1800						364	256	199
50	900				211	175	150	132	118
50	1200				320	241	196	166	145
50	1500					395	284	225	187
50	1800							351	266
60	900				272	221	187	164	146
60	1200					313	249	208	180
60	1500						374	288	236
60	1800								345

Values in table: time in days to lose weight indicated.

WEIGHT LOSS CALORIE TABLE

Sex: Female Height: 4' 11"—5' 5"
Age: 56–75 Yrs. Activity Level 2

WT. LOSS	DIET CALORIES	PRESENT WEIGHT LBS.							
		110	120	130	140	160	180	200	220
5	900	18	16	15	14	12	10	9	8
5	1200	26	22	20	18	15	13	11	10
5	1500	44	35	29	25	19	16	14	12
5	1800	140	77	53	41	28	21	17	15
10	900	38	34	31	28	25	22	19	18
10	1200	54	47	41	37	31	26	23	20
10	1500	95	74	61	52	40	33	28	25
10	1800	385	177	117	88	59	45	36	30
15	900		53	48	44	38	33	30	27
15	1200		73	64	57	47	40	35	31
15	1500		118	96	81	63	51	43	38
15	1800		318	194	142	93	70	56	47
20	900		73	66	60	51	45	40	36
20	1200		102	88	78	64	55	48	43
20	1500		169	135	113	86	70	59	51
20	1800			294	205	130	96	77	64
30	900			104	95	80	70	62	56
30	1200			143	126	102	86	75	66
30	1500			231	188	139	111	93	80
30	1800				382	218	156	122	101
40	900				133	112	97	86	77
40	1200				181	143	120	103	91
40	1500				283	200	157	129	111
40	1800					336	227	173	141
50	900				177	147	126	111	99
50	1200				246	191	157	134	118
50	1500					275	209	170	144
50	1800						315	233	187
60	900				227	185	157	138	123
60	1200				328	245	199	168	146
60	1500					370	270	216	181
60	1800							304	238

Values in table: time in days to lose weight indicated.

WEIGHT LOSS CALORIE TABLE

Sex: Female Height: 4′ 11″—5′ 5″
Age: 56–75 Yrs. Activity Level 3

WT. LOSS	DIET CALORIES	PRESENT WEIGHT LBS.							
		110	120	130	140	160	180	200	220
5	900	14	13	12	11	9	8	7	7
5	1200	19	16	15	13	11	10	8	8
5	1500	27	23	19	17	14	11	10	9
5	1800	47	35	28	23	18	14	12	10
10	900	30	27	25	23	20	17	15	14
10	1200	40	35	31	28	23	20	18	16
10	1500	57	48	41	36	29	24	21	18
10	1800	105	76	60	49	37	30	25	21
15	900		42	38	35	30	26	24	21
15	1200		54	48	43	36	31	27	24
15	1500		75	64	55	44	37	32	28
15	1800		124	95	78	57	46	38	33
20	900		58	52	48	41	36	32	29
20	1200		75	66	59	49	42	37	33
20	1500		105	89	77	61	50	43	38
20	1800		181	136	110	80	63	52	44
30	900			83	75	64	56	50	45
30	1200			106	94	77	66	57	51
30	1500			147	125	97	79	68	59
30	1800			242	186	130	100	82	70
40	900				106	89	78	69	62
40	1200				134	108	91	79	70
40	1500				183	138	111	94	81
40	1800				291	190	143	115	97
50	900				140	117	101	89	79
50	1200				181	143	120	103	91
50	1500				256	186	148	123	106
50	1800					266	193	153	127
60	900				180	147	126	110	98
60	1200				237	183	151	129	113
60	1500				357	244	189	155	132
60	1800					372	253	195	160

Values in table: time in days to lose weight indicated.

WEIGHT LOSS CALORIE TABLE

Sex: Female Height: 5′ 6″—6′ 0″
Age: 18–35 Yrs. Activity Level 0

WT. LOSS	DIET CALORIES	PRESENT WEIGHT LBS.							
		130	140	150	160	180	200	220	240
5	900	16	14	13	13	11	10	9	9
5	1200	21	19	17	16	14	12	11	10
5	1500	31	27	24	22	18	15	14	12
5	1800	63	48	39	33	25	21	17	15
10	900	32	30	28	26	23	21	19	18
10	1200	43	39	36	33	29	25	23	21
10	1500	66	57	50	45	37	32	28	25
10	1800	137	103	83	69	53	43	36	31
20	900		63	58	55	49	44	40	37
20	1200		83	76	69	60	53	48	43
20	1500		124	108	95	78	67	58	52
20	1800		241	186	152	113	91	76	66
30	900			91	85	75	68	62	57
30	1200			120	109	94	82	74	67
30	1500			174	153	124	105	91	81
30	1800			324	256	183	144	119	102
40	900				118	104	93	84	77
40	1200				153	130	113	101	91
40	1500				220	174	146	126	111
40	1800				394	266	204	167	142
50	900					134	120	108	99
50	1200					170	147	130	117
50	1500					232	191	164	144
50	1800					369	274	220	185
60	900					167	148	133	122
60	1200					214	183	161	145
60	1500					298	242	205	178
60	1800						357	280	233
70	900						178	160	146
70	1200						223	195	174
70	1500						299	250	216
70	1800							350	286

Values in table: time in days to lose weight indicated.

WEIGHT LOSS CALORIE TABLE

Sex: Female Height: 5′ 6″—6′ 0″
Age: 18–35 Yrs. Activity Level 1

WT. LOSS	DIET CALORIES	PRESENT WEIGHT LBS.							
		130	140	150	160	180	200	220	240
5	900	14	13	12	12	10	9	9	8
5	1200	19	17	16	15	13	11	10	9
5	1500	27	24	21	19	16	14	12	11
5	1800	48	39	32	28	22	18	15	13
10	900	30	28	26	24	22	20	18	17
10	1200	39	36	33	30	26	23	21	19
10	1500	57	50	44	40	33	29	25	23
10	1800	104	82	68	58	45	37	32	28
20	900		58	54	51	45	41	37	34
20	1200		76	69	63	55	48	43	40
20	1500		108	94	84	70	60	52	47
20	1800		186	150	126	96	78	66	57
30	900			85	79	70	63	57	53
30	1200			109	100	85	75	67	61
30	1500			152	135	110	93	82	73
30	1800			255	208	154	124	104	90
40	900				110	96	86	78	72
40	1200				140	119	104	92	84
40	1500				192	155	130	113	100
40	1800				313	222	175	145	124
50	900					125	111	100	92
50	1200					155	134	119	107
50	1500					205	170	146	129
50	1800					305	233	190	162
60	900					155	137	124	113
60	1200					195	168	148	132
60	1500					263	215	183	160
60	1800						301	241	203
70	900						166	149	135
70	1200						204	178	159
70	1500						265	223	194
70	1800						383	300	248

Values in table: time in days to lose weight indicated.

WEIGHT LOSS CALORIE TABLE

Sex: Female Height: 5′ 6″—6′ 0″
Age: 18–35 Yrs. Activity Level 2

WT. LOSS	DIET CALORIES	PRESENT WEIGHT LBS.							
		130	140	150	160	180	200	220	240
5	900	12	12	11	10	9	8	7	7
5	1200	16	14	13	12	11	9	8	8
5	1500	21	19	17	15	13	11	10	9
5	1800	32	27	23	20	16	14	12	10
10	900	26	24	22	21	19	17	15	14
10	1200	33	30	27	25	22	19	18	16
10	1500	44	39	35	32	27	23	20	18
10	1800	68	56	48	42	34	28	25	22
20	900		50	47	44	39	35	32	29
20	1200		63	57	53	46	41	37	33
20	1500		84	74	67	56	48	43	38
20	1800		124	105	91	72	60	51	45
30	900			73	68	60	54	49	45
30	1200			91	83	72	63	56	51
30	1500			119	106	88	76	66	59
30	1800			173	147	114	94	80	70
40	900				95	83	74	67	62
40	1200				116	99	87	78	70
40	1500				151	123	105	92	81
40	1800				215	163	132	112	97
50	900					108	96	86	79
50	1200					130	113	100	90
50	1500					163	137	119	105
50	1800					220	175	146	126
60	900					134	119	107	97
60	1200					163	140	124	111
60	1500					207	172	148	130
60	1800					288	223	184	157
70	900						143	128	116
70	1200						171	150	134
70	1500						212	180	157
70	1800						280	226	191

Values in table: time in days to lose weight indicated.

WEIGHT LOSS CALORIE TABLE

Sex: Female Height: 5′ 6″—6′ 0″
Age: 18–35 Yrs. Activity Level 3

WT. LOSS	DIET CALORIES	PRESENT WEIGHT LBS.							
		130	140	150	160	180	200	220	240
5	900	10	9	9	8	7	7	6	5
5	1200	12	11	10	10	8	7	7	6
5	1500	15	14	12	11	10	8	8	7
5	1800	21	18	16	14	12	10	9	8
10	900	21	20	18	17	15	14	12	11
10	1200	26	23	22	20	17	15	14	13
10	1500	32	29	26	24	20	18	16	14
10	1800	44	37	33	29	24	21	18	16
20	900		42	39	36	32	29	26	24
20	1200		50	45	42	37	32	29	26
20	1500		62	55	50	43	37	33	30
20	1800		82	71	63	51	44	38	34
30	900			60	56	50	44	40	37
30	1200			72	66	57	50	45	41
30	1500			88	80	67	58	51	46
30	1800			115	101	81	68	59	52
40	900				78	68	61	55	51
40	1200				92	79	69	62	56
40	1500				113	94	80	71	63
40	1800				145	115	95	82	72
50	900					89	79	71	65
50	1200					103	90	80	72
50	1500					123	105	91	81
50	1800					153	125	107	93
60	900					110	98	88	80
60	1200					129	112	99	89
60	1500					156	131	114	101
60	1800					197	159	134	116
70	900						118	105	95
70	1200						136	119	107
70	1500						161	138	122
70	1800						197	164	141

Values in table: time in days to lose weight indicated.

WEIGHT LOSS CALORIE TABLE

Sex: Female Height: 5' 6"—6' 0"
Age: 36–55 Yrs. Activity Level 0

WT. LOSS	DIET CALORIES	PRESENT WEIGHT LBS.							
		130	140	150	160	180	200	220	240
5	900	17	16	15	14	12	11	10	9
5	1200	23	21	19	18	15	13	12	11
5	1500	37	32	28	24	20	17	15	13
5	1800	89	63	49	40	30	24	20	17
10	900	35	32	30	28	25	23	21	19
10	1200	49	44	40	36	31	28	25	22
10	1500	78	66	57	51	42	35	31	27
10	1800	204	137	104	85	62	49	41	35
20	900		68	63	59	52	47	43	39
20	1200		93	84	76	65	57	51	46
20	1500		145	124	109	88	74	64	57
20	1800		341	242	189	133	104	85	73
30	900			99	92	81	72	66	60
30	1200			133	120	102	89	79	71
30	1500			203	175	139	116	100	88
30	1800				327	218	166	135	114
40	900				127	111	99	90	82
40	1200				169	142	123	109	98
40	1500				254	197	162	138	121
40	1800					323	238	190	159
50	900					144	128	115	105
50	1200					186	160	141	126
50	1500					264	213	180	157
50	1800						323	252	208
60	900						158	142	129
60	1200						200	175	156
60	1500						271	226	196
60	1800							324	263
70	900						191	171	155
70	1200						244	211	187
70	1500						338	278	238
70	1800								325

Values in table: time in days to lose weight indicated.

WEIGHT LOSS CALORIE TABLE

Sex: Female Height: 5' 6"—6' 0"
Age: 36–55 Yrs. Activity Level 1

WT. LOSS	DIET CALORIES	PRESENT WEIGHT LBS.							
		130	140	150	160	180	200	220	240
5	900	16	14	13	13	11	10	9	8
5	1200	21	19	17	16	14	12	11	10
5	1500	32	27	24	21	18	15	13	12
5	1800	63	48	38	32	25	20	17	15
10	900	32	30	28	26	23	21	19	17
10	1200	44	39	36	33	28	25	22	20
10	1500	66	57	50	44	37	31	27	24
10	1800	138	102	82	68	51	41	35	30
20	900		63	58	54	48	43	39	36
20	1200		83	75	69	59	52	46	42
20	1500		124	107	95	77	65	57	51
20	1800		241	184	150	110	88	73	63
30	900			91	85	74	67	61	56
30	1200			119	109	92	81	72	65
30	1500			174	152	122	102	89	78
30	1800			323	253	179	140	115	98
40	900				118	103	92	83	76
40	1200				153	129	112	99	89
40	1500				219	172	143	123	108
40	1800				392	261	199	162	137
50	900					133	118	106	97
50	1200					168	145	128	115
50	1500					229	188	160	140
50	1800					364	267	213	179
60	900					166	146	131	120
60	1200					212	181	159	142
60	1500					296	238	200	174
60	1800						349	272	225
70	900						177	158	143
70	1200						221	192	170
70	1500						295	245	211
70	1800							341	277

Values in table: time in days to lose weight indicated.

WEIGHT LOSS CALORIE TABLE

Sex: Female Height: 5' 6"—6' 0"
Age: 36–55 Yrs. Activity Level 2

WT. LOSS	DIET CALORIES	PRESENT WEIGHT LBS.							
		130	140	150	160	180	200	220	240
5	900	13	12	11	11	9	8	8	7
5	1200	17	15	14	13	11	10	9	8
5	1500	24	21	18	17	14	12	11	9
5	1800	38	31	26	23	18	15	13	11
10	900	28	26	24	22	20	18	16	15
10	1200	35	32	29	27	23	21	19	17
10	1500	49	43	38	34	29	25	22	20
10	1800	81	65	55	47	37	31	27	23
20	900		54	50	46	41	37	33	31
20	1200		68	62	57	49	43	39	35
20	1500		93	82	73	61	52	46	41
20	1800		146	120	102	80	65	56	48
30	900			78	72	64	57	52	47
30	1200			98	89	76	67	60	54
30	1500			132	117	96	81	71	63
30	1800			201	168	127	103	87	75
40	900				101	88	78	71	65
40	1200				125	106	93	82	74
40	1500				166	134	113	98	87
40	1800				249	182	145	121	105
50	900					114	101	91	83
50	1200					139	120	106	95
50	1500					178	148	127	112
50	1800					248	193	159	136
60	900					142	125	112	102
60	1200					175	150	132	118
60	1500					228	187	159	139
60	1800					329	248	201	170
70	900						151	135	122
70	1200						182	159	142
70	1500						230	194	168
70	1800						314	249	208

Values in table: time in days to lose weight indicated.

WEIGHT LOSS CALORIE TABLE

Sex: Female   Height: 5′ 6″—6′ 0″
Age: 36–55 Yrs.   Activity Level 3

WT. LOSS	DIET CALORIES	PRESENT WEIGHT LBS.							
		130	140	150	160	180	200	220	240
5	900	11	10	9	9	8	7	6	6
5	1200	13	12	11	10	9	8	7	6
5	1500	17	15	13	12	10	9	8	7
5	1800	23	20	17	15	12	11	9	8
10	900	22	21	19	18	16	14	13	12
10	1200	27	25	23	21	18	16	15	13
10	1500	35	31	28	25	22	19	17	15
10	1800	49	41	36	32	26	22	19	17
20	900		44	41	38	33	30	27	25
20	1200		53	48	44	38	34	30	28
20	1500		67	60	54	45	39	35	31
20	1800		90	78	68	55	46	40	35
30	900			63	59	52	46	42	38
30	1200			76	70	60	53	47	43
30	1500			95	85	71	61	54	48
30	1800			127	110	88	73	63	55
40	900				82	72	64	58	53
40	1200				98	83	73	65	59
40	1500				121	100	85	74	66
40	1800				159	124	102	87	76
50	900					93	82	74	67
50	1200					109	94	84	75
50	1500					131	111	96	85
50	1800					166	134	114	99
60	900					116	102	91	83
60	1200					137	118	104	93
60	1500					167	139	120	106
60	1800					215	171	143	123
70	900						123	110	99
70	1200						143	125	112
70	1500						171	146	128
70	1800						213	175	150

Values in table: time in days to lose weight indicated.

WEIGHT LOSS CALORIE TABLE

Sex: Female Height: 5' 6"—6' 0"
Age: 56–75 Yrs. Activity Level 0

WT. LOSS	DIET CALORIES	PRESENT WEIGHT LBS.							
		130	140	150	160	180	200	220	240
5	900	18	17	16	15	13	12	11	10
5	1200	26	23	21	19	16	14	13	12
5	1500	44	37	32	28	22	19	16	14
5	1800	146	88	63	49	35	27	22	19
10	900	38	35	32	30	27	24	22	20
10	1200	54	48	43	40	34	30	26	24
10	1500	94	78	66	58	46	39	34	30
10	1800	367	198	137	105	73	56	46	39
20	900		73	68	63	55	50	45	41
20	1200		103	92	84	71	62	55	50
20	1500		172	144	124	98	82	70	62
20	1800			335	243	159	120	96	81
30	900			106	98	86	77	70	64
30	1200			147	132	111	96	85	77
30	1500			239	202	156	128	109	96
30	1800					265	193	153	127
40	900				137	119	106	95	87
40	1200				187	155	133	117	105
40	1500				297	223	180	152	132
40	1800						279	217	178
50	900					154	136	123	112
50	1200					204	173	152	135
50	1500					301	238	199	171
50	1800						385	290	234
60	900					193	169	151	137
60	1200					258	217	189	167
60	1500					396	305	251	214
60	1800							376	298
70	900						205	182	164
70	1200						266	229	202
70	1500						383	309	261
70	1800								371

Values in table: time in days to lose weight indicated.

WEIGHT LOSS CALORIE TABLE

Sex: Female   Height: 5' 6"—6' 0"
Age: 56–75 Yrs.   Activity Level 1

WT. LOSS	DIET CALORIES	PRESENT WEIGHT LBS.							
		130	140	150	160	180	200	220	240
5	900	17	15	14	13	12	11	10	9
5	1200	23	21	19	17	15	13	12	10
5	1500	37	31	27	24	19	16	14	13
5	1800	86	61	47	38	28	22	19	16
10	900	35	32	30	28	25	22	20	18
10	1200	48	43	39	36	30	27	24	22
10	1500	77	65	56	49	40	34	30	26
10	1800	197	132	100	81	59	46	39	33
20	900		67	62	58	51	46	41	38
20	1200		92	82	75	64	56	50	45
20	1500		143	122	106	85	71	62	54
20	1800		330	233	182	127	99	81	69
30	900			98	90	79	71	64	59
30	1200			131	118	100	87	77	69
30	1500			199	172	135	112	96	84
30	1800				314	209	158	128	108
40	900				126	109	97	88	80
40	1200				167	139	120	106	95
40	1500				249	192	157	133	116
40	1800					310	227	181	151
50	900					142	125	113	103
50	1200					183	156	137	122
50	1500					257	207	174	151
50	1800						308	240	198
60	900					177	156	139	126
60	1200					231	195	170	151
60	1500					335	263	219	188
60	1800							309	250
70	900						188	167	151
70	1200						239	206	182
70	1500						329	269	229
70	1800							390	310

Values in table: time in days to lose weight indicated.

WEIGHT LOSS CALORIE TABLE

Sex: Female Height: 5' 6"—6' 0"
Age: 56–75 Yrs. Activity Level 2

WT. LOSS	DIET CALORIES	PRESENT WEIGHT LBS.							
		130	140	150	160	180	200	220	240
5	900	14	13	12	11	10	9	8	7
5	1200	18	17	15	14	12	11	9	9
5	1500	26	23	20	18	15	13	11	10
5	1800	45	36	30	25	20	16	14	12
10	900	29	27	25	23	21	19	17	15
10	1200	38	35	31	29	25	22	20	18
10	1500	55	48	42	37	31	27	23	21
10	1800	97	76	63	53	41	34	29	25
20	900		57	53	49	43	39	35	32
20	1200		74	67	61	52	46	41	37
20	1500		103	90	80	65	56	49	43
20	1800		174	139	116	88	71	60	52
30	900			83	77	67	60	54	50
30	1200			105	96	81	71	63	57
30	1500			146	128	103	87	76	67
30	1800			237	193	142	113	94	81
40	900				107	93	82	74	68
40	1200				135	113	98	87	78
40	1500				184	146	122	105	92
40	1800				291	205	160	132	112
50	900					120	106	95	87
50	1200					148	128	112	100
50	1500					194	160	136	119
50	1800					281	214	173	147
60	900					150	132	118	107
60	1200					187	160	139	124
60	1500					250	202	171	148
60	1800					379	277	220	184
70	900						160	142	128
70	1200						195	169	150
70	1500						250	209	180
70	1800						353	274	226

Values in table: time in days to lose weight indicated.

WEIGHT LOSS CALORIE TABLE

Sex: Female Height: 5' 6"—6' 0"
Age: 56-75 Yrs. Activity Level 3

WT. LOSS	DIET CALORIES	PRESENT WEIGHT LBS.							
		130	140	150	160	180	200	220	240
5	900	11	10	10	9	8	7	6	6
5	1200	14	13	12	11	9	8	7	7
5	1500	18	16	14	13	11	9	8	7
5	1800	26	22	19	16	13	11	10	9
10	900	24	22	20	19	17	15	14	12
10	1200	29	26	24	22	19	17	15	14
10	1500	38	33	30	27	23	20	17	16
10	1800	54	45	39	34	28	23	20	18
20	900		46	42	40	35	31	28	26
20	1200		56	51	47	40	36	32	29
20	1500		72	64	57	48	41	36	32
20	1800		100	85	74	59	49	42	37
30	900			67	62	54	48	44	40
30	1200			81	74	63	55	49	44
30	1500			102	91	76	65	57	50
30	1800			140	120	94	78	66	58
40	900				86	75	66	60	54
40	1200				103	88	76	68	61
40	1500				130	106	90	78	69
40	1800				175	134	109	92	80
50	900					97	86	77	70
50	1200					115	99	88	79
50	1500					140	117	101	90
50	1800					180	144	121	104
60	900					121	106	95	86
60	1200					144	124	109	97
60	1500					178	148	127	111
60	1800					235	184	152	130
70	900						129	114	103
70	1200						151	131	117
70	1500						182	154	134
70	1800						230	187	159

Values in table: time in days to lose weight indicated.

6. Weight Loss Diet Tables

At this point, the weight loss caloric values discussed previously will be translated into practical eating guidelines. My purpose is to make it as easy as possible for you to account for the calories contained in the meals you eat. With this in mind, another group of tables, which I call Weight Loss Diet Tables, were produced on a digital computer. Each diet table represents a *complete* meal type.

The tables are general in nature and do not specify any particular recipe. But each table does represent a particular meal type and indicates the total caloric value which results when certain food combinations and portion sizes are eaten. The general nature of the tables was arrived at by averaging the caloric content of foods within the same group. For example, I allowed 50 calories for a piece of fresh fruit because this was the approximate calculated average for all fruit portions.

How to Use the Diet Tables

The use of the Weight Loss Diet Tables is relatively straightforward. However, one point does require an explanation. If you scan the Weight Loss Diet Tables that begin on page 110, you will find beverage types designated as A, B, C, or D (there is a similar designation for desserts). Since there are so many different kinds of beverages (and desserts), I have grouped together those that have the same approximate calorie content. This was done in order to allow you maximum latitude in choosing the particular type of beverage (or dessert) you prefer and to keep the size of each diet table within reasonable bounds. You should use the table headed Beverage and Dessert Type Designation to determine the particular beverages (or desserts) that correspond to a given letter designation. For example, when any of the Weight Loss Diet Tables indicates a

BEVERAGE AND DESSERT TYPE DESIGNATION

TYPE	BEVERAGE DESCRIPTION
A	Water, black coffee or tea (no sugar), non-caloric soft drink.
B	Regular coffee or tea (1 ounce milk, 1 tsp. sugar), 4 ounces skim milk.
C	8 ounces skim milk, 4 ounces whole milk, 4 ounces wine, 8 ounces apple cider.
D	8 ounces whole milk, 12-ounce can of beer or soft drink, 4 ounces wine, cup of regular coffee.
TYPE	DESSERT DESCRIPTION
A	Small apple, 3 apricots, 1/2 cantaloupe melon, 1/2 cup cherries, one fig, 1/2 grapefruit, one cup grapes, orange, large peach, one cup strawberries, tangerine.
B	Flavored gelatin, angel food cake, donut, 3 cookies, fruit cup, plain cake (no icing).
C	Flavored yogurt (cup), iced layer cake, cup of ice cream or sherbet.
D	Cheese cake, pastry, pie, baked custard (cup).

type A beverage, you can choose from water, black coffee, or tea (without sugar), or a non-caloric soft drink.

As you can see from the Weight Loss Diet Table Index on page 109, there are eleven tables in all. Each table carries an alpha-numeric designation such as DB-1 (which in this case refers to *D*iet *B*reakfast number *1*). The value of the diet tables is threefold.

1. They can be used to determine the number of calories in a given meal. For example, to find the number of calories in a breakfast of: 4 ounces of juice, a soft-boiled egg, buttered toast, and a cup of coffee with an ounce of milk and a teaspoon of sugar—designated as beverage type B and labeled regular coffee in the tables—you proceed as follows. Using the Weight Loss Diet Table Index, you identify this food combination as meal type DB-1. The Index shows that the table for meal DB-1 is on page 110. On page 110, you find that the exact food combination given in the example is the fifth one listed (the fifth horizontal line) on the table and has a calorie total of 280.
2. The tables can also be used to get an idea of the kind of food you may eat on your diet and what the permissible portion sizes are. Let's assume your particular diet allows 500 calories for breakfast and your favorite breakfast consists of eggs and cereal. Meal type DB-3 shows that 6 ounces of juice, one cup of cereal, a poached egg, a strip of bacon, one slice of buttered toast, and a cup of coffee with milk and sugar totals 490 calories (the twelfth horizontal line). Quite a substantial breakfast, and yet permitted on this particular diet.
3. Perhaps the most important use of the tables will be when you plan your personal diet menu. An ex-

ample of this is shown in Appendix A. The 7-day diets of 900, 1200, 1500, 1800 and 2100 calories per day were devised by using the Weight Loss Diet Tables.

Additional Notes About the Diet Tables

The Weight Loss Diet Tables are designed to be as self-contained as possible; however, the following notes are intended to expand and clarify certain information in the tables.

1. In the breakfast tables, in place of juice you may substitute any of the fresh fruit portions listed as a type A dessert. Try to use those high in vitamin C, such as ½ cantaloupe melon, ½ grapefruit, an orange, or a cup of strawberries.
2. Since the calorie count of most commercially available cereals is approximately the same, you may use any unsweetened brand where cereal is indicated.
3. Where bacon is indicated, you may substitute one ounce of ham (usually this amounts to one thin slice) or one ounce of sausage for two strips of bacon.
4. Fried eggs are acceptable if they are prepared without fat or butter (in a Teflon-lined pan, for example).
5. Add 40 to the calorie total if a second cup of coffee or tea with milk and sugar is taken.
6. In the lunch and dinner tables, permitted fresh or cooked vegetables include: asparagus, green or wax beans, beets, broccoli, brussels sprouts, cabbage, carrots, cauliflower, collards, cucumbers, dandelion, kale, mushrooms, onions, peppers, radish, spinach,

summer squash, tomatoes, and turnips. (No butter is to be added to vegetables.)
7. Meat and poultry not permitted are: all types of pork, corned beef, pastrami, duck, goose, and the dark meat of chicken and turkey.
8. Try a low calorie salad dressing prepared by mixing one cup of tomato juice with 3 tbsp. of vinegar or lemon juice; season to taste with onion flakes, parsley, salt, and pepper.
9. Where meat is indicated, it is assumed to be cooked, lean, and trimmed of all fat.

Again, remember that men (and women past menopause) should avoid butter and bacon.

The food values in the diet tables are based on averages. If you are reasonable and use judgment, these tables can be a very useful new diet tool.

Diet Snacks

When dieting, you have a limited amount of food from which to obtain essential nutrients. Sensible snacking can help you meet your nutritional needs while soothing those hunger pangs. But indiscriminate eating between meals usually leads to more calories than are wanted—and fewer nutrients than are needed. Snacks are important. The following is a list of snacks of varying calorie content, which I have grouped into four categories:

1. Zero-calorie snacks(*): Cup of bouillon, celery sticks, black coffee or tea (no sugar), green salad (no dressing), and non-caloric soft drink.

* No significant calories.

2. Low-calorie (50): Choose any of the fresh fruits listed as type A in the Beverage and Dessert Type Designation Table or a plain cookie, 4 ounces of skim milk, or coffee or tea with milk and sugar.
3. Mid-calorie (100): Choose a banana, buttered toast, 8 ounces of skim milk, or 2 plain cookies.
4. High-calorie (150): Choose either ½ cup of flavored yogurt, ice cream, or creamed cottage cheese on lettuce.

If you don't see your favorite snack, look it up in a calorie chart and add it to the list.

WEIGHT LOSS DIET TABLE INDEX

MEAL	BASIS	TYPE	PAGE NO.
Breakfast	Eggs	DB-1	110
	Cereal	DB-2	111
	Eggs and Cereal	DB-3	112
Lunch	Meat or Poultry	DL-1	113
	Fish	DL-2	114
	Tuna (in water)	DL-3	115
	Tuna (oil)	DL-4	116
	Uncreamed Cottage Cheese	DL-5	117
	Creamed Cottage Cheese	DL-6	118
Dinner	Meat or Poultry	DD-1	119
	Fish	DD-2	120

WEIGHT LOSS DIET TABLE

Meal: Breakfast   Type: DB-1

Content: Juice or Fresh Fruit
Eggs, Soft-Boiled or Poached
Crisp Bacon or Equivalent
Toast, Beverage

Calorie Total	Eggs	Juice Oz.	Toast Slices	Bacon Strips	Beverage Type
210	1	4	*	0	A
250	1	4	*	0	B
290	1	4	*	0	2-B
240	1	4	1	0	A
280	1	4	1	0	B
320	1	4	1	0	2-B
270	1	4	1	1	A
310	1	4	1	1	B
350	1	4	1	1	2-B
310	1	4	1	2	A
350	1	4	1	2	B
390	1	4	1	2	2-B
340	1	6	1	2	A
380	1	6	1	2	B
420	1	6	1	2	2-B
310	2	4	1	0	A
350	2	4	1	0	B
390	2	4	1	0	2-B
410	2	4	2	0	A
450	2	4	2	0	B
490	2	4	2	0	2-B
480	2	4	2	2	A
520	2	4	2	2	B
560	2	4	2	2	2-B
510	2	6	2	2	A
550	2	6	2	2	B
590	2	6	2	2	2-B

If toast is designated * (plain), use no butter. Otherwise a maximum of ½ pat of butter or margarine per slice of toast is permitted. Bacon is to be free of excess oil or grease (pat dry).

WEIGHT LOSS DIET TABLE

Meal: Breakfast   Type: DB-2

Content: Juice or Fresh Fruit
Hot or Cold Cereal
Skim Milk
Fruit for Cereal
Beverage

Calorie Total	Juice Oz.	Cereal Cups	Milk Oz.	Fruit Cups	Beverage Type
210	4	1	5	0	A
250	4	1	5	0	B
280	4	1	5	1/2	A
320	4	1	5	1/2	B
240	6	1	5	0	A
280	6	1	5	0	B
310	6	1	5	1/2	A
350	6	1	5	1/2	B
350	4	2	10	0	A
390	4	2	10	0	B
420	4	2	10	1	A
460	4	2	10	1	B
380	6	2	10	0	A
420	6	2	10	0	B
450	6	2	10	1	A
490	6	2	10	1	B

Do not use sugar in cereal.

WEIGHT LOSS DIET TABLE

Meal: Breakfast Type: DB-3

Content: Juice or Fresh Fruit
Cereal with Skim Milk
Eggs, Soft-Boiled or Poached
Crisp Bacon or Equivalent
Beverage

Calorie Total	Juice Oz.	Cereal Cups	Eggs	Bacon Strips	Toast Slices	Beverage Type
290	4	1	1	0	0	A
330	4	1	1	0	0	B
350	4	1	1	0	*	A
390	4	1	1	0	*	B
380	4	1	1	0	1	A
420	4	1	1	0	1	B
420	4	1	1	1	1	A
460	4	1	1	1	1	B
410	6	1	1	0	1	A
450	6	1	1	0	1	B
450	6	1	1	1	1	A
490	6	1	1	1	1	B
370	4	1	2	0	0	A
410	4	1	2	0	0	B
430	4	1	2	0	*	A
470	4	1	2	0	*	B
460	4	1	2	0	1	A
500	4	1	2	0	1	B
500	4	1	2	1	1	A
540	4	1	2	1	1	B
490	6	1	2	0	1	A
530	6	1	2	0	1	B
530	6	1	2	1	1	A
570	6	1	2	1	1	B

Use no more than 5 ounces of skim milk and no sugar in cereal. If toast is designated * (plain), use no butter. Otherwise a maximum of ½ pat of butter or margarine per slice of toast is permitted. Bacon is to be free of excess oil or grease (pat dry).

WEIGHT LOSS DIET TABLE

Meal: Lunch   Type: DL-1
Content: Broiled Lean Meat, or Poultry
Fresh or Cooked Vegetables
Green Salad
Bread, Beverage, and Dessert

Calorie Total	Meat Oz.	Vegetable Cups	Bread Slices	Beverage Type	Dessert Type
170	2	1/2	0	A	None
170	2	0	0	A	A
210	2	1/2	0	B	None
210	2	0	0	B	A
230	2	1/2	1	A	None
230	2	0	1	A	A
270	2	1/2	1	B	None
270	2	0	1	B	A
320	2	1/2	1	B	A
290	4	1/2	0	A	None
290	4	0	0	A	A
330	4	1/2	0	B	None
330	4	0	0	B	A
350	4	1/2	1	A	None
350	4	0	1	A	A
390	4	1/2	1	B	None
390	4	0	1	B	A
440	4	1/2	1	B	A
410	6	1/2	0	A	None
410	6	0	0	A	A
450	6	1/2	0	B	None
450	6	0	0	B	A
470	6	1/2	1	A	None
470	6	0	1	A	A
510	6	1/2	1	B	None
510	6	0	1	B	A
560	6	1/2	1	B	A

Do not use butter or margarine on bread. As a guide to judging meat portion size, a slice of meat 4 × 4 × ⅛ inch weighs approximately 2 ounces. An unlimited amount of green salad may be eaten without significantly increasing the calorie totals.

WEIGHT LOSS DIET TABLE

Meal: Lunch   Type: DL-2
Content: Broiled Fish
          Fresh or Cooked Vegetables
          Green Salad
          Bread, Beverage, and Dessert

Calorie Total	Fish Oz.	Vegetable Cups	Bread Slices	Beverage Type	Dessert Type
130	2	1/2	0	A	None
130	2	0	0	A	A
170	2	1/2	0	B	None
170	2	0	0	B	A
190	2	1/2	1	A	None
190	2	0	1	A	A
230	2	1/2	1	B	None
230	2	0	1	B	A
280	2	1/2	1	B	A
210	4	1/2	0	A	None
210	4	0	0	A	A
250	4	1/2	0	B	None
250	4	0	0	B	A
270	4	1/2	1	A	None
270	4	0	1	A	A
310	4	1/2	1	B	None
310	4	0	1	B	A
360	4	1/2	1	B	A
290	6	1/2	0	A	None
290	6	0	0	A	A
330	6	1/2	0	B	None
330	6	0	0	B	A
350	6	1/2	1	A	None
350	6	0	1	A	A
390	6	1/2	1	B	None
390	6	0	1	B	A
440	6	1/2	1	B	A

Broil fish without using added fat or butter. Do not use butter or margarine on bread. An unlimited amount of green salad may be eaten without significantly increasing the calorie totals. No butter or margarine is to be added to vegetables.

WEIGHT LOSS DIET TABLE

Meal: Lunch   Type: DL-3
Content: Tuna (Canned in Water)
          Fresh or Cooked Vegetables
          Green Salad
          Bread, Beverage, and Dessert

Calorie Total	Tuna Oz.	Vegetable Cups	Bread Slices	Beverage Type	Dessert Type
120	2	1/2	0	A	None
120	2	0	0	A	A
160	2	1/2	0	B	None
160	2	0	0	B	A
180	2	1/2	1	A	None
180	2	0	1	A	A
220	2	1/2	1	B	None
220	2	0	1	B	A
270	2	1/2	1	B	A
190	4	1/2	0	A	None
190	4	0	0	A	A
230	4	1/2	0	B	None
230	4	0	0	B	A
250	4	1/2	1	A	None
250	4	0	1	A	A
290	4	1/2	1	B	None
290	4	0	1	B	A
340	4	1/2	1	B	A
260	6	1/2	0	A	None
260	6	0	0	A	A
300	6	1/2	0	B	None
300	6	0	0	B	A
320	6	1/2	0	A	None
320	6	0	1	A	A
360	6	1/2	1	B	None
360	6	0	1	B	A
410	6	1/2	1	B	A

Do not use butter or margarine on bread. An unlimited amount of green salad may be eaten without significantly increasing the calorie totals. No butter or margarine is to be added to vegetables.

WEIGHT LOSS DIET TABLE

Meal: Lunch   Type: DL-4
Content: Tuna (Canned in Oil)
           Fresh or Cooked Vegetables
           Green Salad
           Bread, Beverage, and Dessert

Calorie Total	Tuna Oz.	Vegetable Cups	Bread Slices	Beverage Type	Dessert Type
160	2	1/2	0	A	None
160	2	0	0	A	A
200	2	1/2	0	B	None
200	2	0	0	B	A
220	2	1/2	1	A	None
220	2	0	1	A	A
260	2	1/2	1	B	None
260	2	0	1	B	A
310	2	1/2	1	B	A
270	4	1/2	0	A	None
270	4	0	0	A	A
310	4	1/2	0	B	None
310	4	0	0	B	A
330	4	1/2	1	A	None
330	4	0	1	A	A
370	4	1/2	1	B	None
370	4	0	1	B	A
420	4	1/2	1	B	A
380	6	1/2	0	A	None
380	6	0	0	A	A
420	6	1/2	0	B	None
420	6	0	0	B	A
440	6	1/2	1	A	None
440	6	0	1	A	A
480	6	1/2	1	B	None
480	6	0	1	B	A
530	6	1/2	1	B	A

Do not use butter or margarine on bread. Tuna must be well drained of oil. An unlimited amount of green salad may be eaten without significantly increasing the calorie totals. No butter or margarine is to be added to vegetables.

WEIGHT LOSS DIET TABLE

Meal: Lunch   Type: DL-5
Content: Uncreamed Cottage Cheese
           Fresh or Cooked Vegetables
           Green Salad
           Bread, Beverage, and Dessert

Calorie Total	Cottage Cheese Cups	Vegetable Cups	Bread Slices	Beverage Type	Dessert Type
140	1/2	1/2	0	A	None
140	1/2	0	0	A	A
180	1/2	1/2	0	B	None
180	1/2	0	0	B	A
200	1/2	1/2	1	A	None
200	1/2	0	1	A	A
260	1/2	1/2	1	B	None
260	1/2	0	1	B	A
310	1/2	1/2	1	B	A
180	3/4	1/2	0	A	None
180	3/4	0	0	A	A
220	3/4	1/2	0	B	None
220	3/4	0	0	B	A
240	3/4	1/2	1	A	None
240	3/4	0	1	A	A
280	3/4	1/2	1	B	None
280	3/4	0	1	B	A
330	3/4	1/2	1	B	A
220	1	1/2	0	A	None
220	1	0	0	A	A
260	1	1/2	0	B	None
260	1	0	0	B	A
280	1	1/2	1	A	None
280	1	0	1	A	A
320	1	1/2	1	B	None
320	1	0	1	B	A
370	1	1/2	1	B	A

Do not use butter or margarine on bread. A substitution of 1½ ounces of hard cheese for a cup of uncreamed cottage cheese will result in approximately the same calorie totals. An unlimited amount of green salad may be eaten without significantly increasing the calorie totals. No butter or margarine is to be added to vegetables.

WEIGHT LOSS DIET TABLE

Meal: Lunch Type: DL-6
Content: Creamed Cottage Cheese
Fresh or Cooked Vegetables
Green Salad
Bread, Beverage, and Dessert

Calorie Total	Cottage Cheese Cups	Vegetable Cups	Bread Slices	Beverage Type	Dessert Type
180	1/2	1/2	0	A	None
180	1/2	0	0	A	A
220	1/2	1/2	0	B	None
220	1/2	0	0	B	A
240	1/2	1/2	1	A	None
240	1/2	0	1	A	A
280	1/2	1/2	1	B	None
280	1/2	0	1	B	A
330	1/2	1/2	1	B	A
250	3/4	1/2	0	A	None
250	3/4	0	0	A	A
290	3/4	1/2	0	B	None
290	3/4	0	0	B	A
310	3/4	1/2	1	A	None
310	3/4	0	1	A	A
350	3/4	1/2	1	B	None
350	3/4	0	1	B	A
400	3/4	1/2	1	B	A
310	1	1/2	0	A	None
310	1	0	0	A	A
350	1	1/2	0	B	None
350	1	0	0	B	A
370	1	1/2	1	A	None
370	1	0	1	A	A
410	1	1/2	1	B	None
410	1	0	1	B	A
460	1	1/2	1	B	A

Do not use butter or margarine on bread. A substitution of 2½ ounces of hard cheese for a cup of creamed cottage cheese will result in approximately the same calorie totals. An unlimited amount of green salad may be eaten without significantly increasing the calorie totals. No butter or margarine is to be added to vegetables.

WEIGHT LOSS DIET TABLE

Meal: Dinner   Type: DD-1
Content: Broiled Lean Meat or Poultry
Fresh or Cooked Vegetables
Green Salad
Bread, Beverage, and Dessert

Calorie Total	Meat Oz.	Vegetable Cups	Bread Slices	Beverage Type	Dessert Type
290	4	1/2	0	A	None
290	4	0	0	A	A
330	4	1/2	0	B	None
330	4	0	0	B	A
350	4	1/2	1	A	None
350	4	0	1	A	A
390	4	1/2	1	B	None
390	4	0	1	B	A
440	4	1/2	1	B	A
540	4	1/2	1	B	B
530	8	1/2	0	A	None
530	8	0	0	A	A
570	8	1/2	0	B	None
570	8	0	0	B	A
590	8	1/2	1	A	None
590	8	0	1	A	A
630	8	1/2	1	B	None
630	8	0	1	B	A
680	8	1/2	1	B	A
780	8	1/2	1	B	B
770	12	1/2	0	A	None
770	12	0	0	A	A
810	12	1/2	0	B	None
810	12	0	0	B	A
830	12	1/2	1	A	None
830	12	0	1	A	A
870	12	1/2	1	B	None
870	12	0	1	B	A
920	12	1/2	1	B	A
1020	12	1/2	1	B	B

Do not use butter or margarine on bread. As a guide to judging meat portion size, a slice of meat 4 x 4 x ⅛ inch weighs approximately 2 ounces. An unlimited amount of green salad may be eaten without significantly increasing the calorie totals. No butter or margarine is to be added to vegetables.

WEIGHT LOSS DIET TABLE

Meal: Dinner Type: DD-2
Content: Broiled Fish
Fresh or Cooked Vegetables
Green Salad
Bread, Beverage, and Dessert

Calorie Total	Fish Oz.	Vegetable Cups	Bread Slices	Beverage Type	Dessert Type
210	4	1/2	0	A	None
210	4	0	0	A	A
250	4	1/2	0	B	None
250	4	0	0	B	A
270	4	1/2	1	A	None
270	4	0	1	A	A
310	4	1/2	1	B	None
310	4	0	1	B	A
360	4	1/2	1	B	A
460	4	1/2	1	B	B
370	8	1/2	0	A	None
370	8	0	0	A	A
410	8	1/2	0	B	None
410	8	0	0	B	A
430	8	1/2	1	A	None
430	8	0	1	A	A
470	8	1/2	1	B	None
470	8	0	1	B	A
520	8	1/2	1	B	A
620	8	1/2	1	B	B
530	12	1/2	0	A	None
530	12	0	0	A	A
570	12	1/2	0	B	None
570	12	0	0	B	A
590	12	1/2	1	A	None
590	12	0	1	A	A
630	12	1/2	1	B	None
630	12	0	1	B	A
680	12	1/2	1	B	A
780	12	1/2	1	B	B

Broil fish without using added fat or butter. Do not use butter or margarine on bread. An unlimited amount of green salad may be eaten without significantly increasing the calorie totals. No butter or margarine is to be added to vegetables.

7. Planning a Weight Loss Program

In the preceding chapters, a great many facts were presented. Now these facts will be pieced together and a logical weight loss program will be developed.

Consider the diet that might be planned by the 32-year-old female described on page 36. As you recall, she wanted to lose fifteen pounds, and her diet options were:

1. 900 calories per day, for 40 days.
2. 1200 calories per day, for 50 days.
3. 1500 calories per day, for 68 days.
4. 1800 calories per day, for 106 days.

In order to lose weight at the recommended rate of not more than two pounds per week, she should lose the fifteen pounds over at least 7½ weeks. Therefore, she should choose diet option 3: 1500 calories per day for 68 days. (Had she chosen diet option 2, 1200 calories for 50 days, she would lose weight at a rate faster than the recommended two pounds per week.) Next she must analyze her eating habits and decide how to spread her caloric allowance—first over the days of the week, and then among the meals of the day.

Weekly Routine: The calorie allowance of a weight loss diet need not be the same for every day of the week so long as the average intake over the entire week equals, in this instance, 1500 calories per day. Let us assume that this dieter's eating habits and social life are such that she invariably eats more on weekends. She could tailor a diet to her needs by deducting 300 calories from her weekday diet and adding this amount to her weekend total. The net result would be a diet of 1200 calories on weekdays, and 2250 calories on weekends. Her average, however, would remain 1500 calories per day, and she would still lose fifteen pounds in 68 days.

Daily Routine: The daily calorie allowance may be divided over the day's meals in accordance with my recommended rule of thumb (divide the total calorie allowance equally among breakfast, lunch, dinner, and your collective in-between-meal snacks) or, if you must, by a scheme more suitable to your eating habits.

Let us consider the 1200 calorie weekday meals. Assume the dieter in our example has chosen to split the day's calories as follows:

Breakfast	300
Mid-morning snack	50
Lunch	300
Dinner	400
Evening snack	150
	1200 calories

She is now ready to use the Weight Loss Diet Tables. The objective in planning any reducing diet should be twofold: First, to restrict caloric intake to the desired level, and second, to plan meals that are nutritionally well balanced and provide all essential nutrients. The Weight Loss Diet Tables allow her to do just that.

The following diet meal combinations are only one set out of many possible patterns she could arrange, which would all result in 1200 calories per day. (To keep this example simple, I am going to restrict the selections to one from each meal type, although in some cases many more are possible.)

Breakfast (300 calories) select from:

DB-1: 4 ounces of juice, one soft boiled egg, buttered toast, one strip of bacon, and coffee with milk and sugar. (310 calories)

DB-2: 4 ounces of juice, 1 cup of cereal with 5 ounces of skim milk, ½ cup of fresh fruit, and coffee with milk and sugar. (320 calories)

Mid-morning snack (50 calories) choose from the low-calorie snacks shown on page 109. Examples are fresh fruit, coffee with milk and sugar, and so on.

Lunch (300 calories) select from:

DL-1: 2 ounces of lean meat or poultry, ½ cup of vegetables, a slice of enriched bread (no butter), 4 ounces of skim milk, and a portion of fresh fruit. (320 calories)

DL-2: 4 ounces of broiled fish, a slice of enriched bread (no butter), 4 ounces of skim milk, and a portion of fresh fruit. (310 calories)

DL-4: 4 ounces of tuna (canned in oil), ½ cup of vegetables, and 4 ounces of skim milk. (310 calories)

DL-6: one cup of creamed cottage cheese, ½ cup of vegetables, and a non-caloric soft drink. (310 calories)

I have arbitrarily limited the choice of tuna to the packed-in-oil variety, and that of cottage cheese to the creamed variety, although the other types shown in

DL-3 and DL-5 could also have been chosen. In addition, remember that you may have an unlimited amount of green salad with any lunch or dinner meal.

Dinner (400 calories) select from:

DD-1: 4 ounces of lean meat or poultry, ½ cup of vegetables, a slice of enriched bread (no butter), and a cup of coffee with milk and sugar. (390 calories)

DD-2: 8 ounces of broiled fish, ½ cup of vegetables, and a cup of coffee with milk and sugar. (410 calories)

Evening snack (150 calories) select either ½ cup of flavored yogurt or ice cream, or 4 ounces of skim milk and 2 plain cookies.

By following the procedure described in this example you will be able to devise your own personalized weight loss eating plan. If you would rather not go through this exercise, I suggest the pre-planned diets in Appendix A. They are especially recommended because they are nutritionally sound.

Of course, when you follow my pre-planned diet, you let *me* tell you exactly what to eat and when. Quite obviously, I have no way of knowing how you would like your caloric allowance allocated over the day's meals—whether you prefer your coffee black or with milk and sugar; if, given a choice, you would select a portion of fresh fruit in place of a cooked vegetable for lunch; and so on. You are the only person who can take these factors into account. So I urge you to follow the previous example and plan your own customized diet menu.

Calorie Control

The advantage of establishing a definite calorie count for each meal is that it is then unnecessary to keep a tally of the total calories for the entire day. Instead, only the number of calories eaten at each meal need be monitored, and there are ways to keep even this to a minimum.

I suggest that you utilize a concept I call Set Meals. By this I mean that certain of the day's meals can be prearranged so as to have an identical calorie count from day to day.

Once again, I ask that you examine your eating habits. Are one or two of the day's meals completely under your control? If so, they are Set Meal candidates. Let's assume you prepare your own breakfast every day. Use the Weight Loss Diet Tables to plan perhaps three set breakfasts. One might be based on eggs and bacon, the second on cereal and fruit, and so on. Variety is obtained by having more than one choice for a Set Meal, and by eating different kinds of cereal or fresh fruit—all within the same Set Meal.

Since you know the calorie content of a Set Meal, you only count calories at the remaining meals. The more Set Meals, the less counting.

Weight Loss Summarized

You now have all the information you need to start a reducing diet. So let's review the procedure you should follow to develop your personal *weight loss plan*.

Step 1. Determine your desirable weight from the table on page 32.

Step 2. Establish your weight loss goal by subtracting your desirable weight from your present weight.
Step 3. Find your Activity Level from the table on page 14.
Step 4. From the Weight Loss Calorie Table Index on page 43, locate the table that applies to you.
Step 5. Use your Weight Loss Calorie Table to determine your four diet options.
Step 6. Choose the diet option best suited to you, and thereby fix your diet duration and caloric intake.
Step 7. Allocate your calorie total among the days of the week.
Step 8. Allocate your calorie allowance among the meals of the day.
Step 9. Consult the Weight Loss Diet Tables (Index on page 109) and choose at least one meal from each of the tables.
Step 10. Determine which of the meals of the day will be Set Meals.

For easy reference, I recommend you record your weekly and daily calorie distribution as well as the ingredients of the meal types you have selected from the Weight Loss Diet Tables. Finally, check to make sure that the meal patterns you choose provide the proper number of servings from the four Essential Food Groups (listed on page 18).

8. Weight Maintenance Calorie Tables

Why do people regain lost weight? In most instances, the reason is that they revert to their pre-dieting eating habits. This cannot be done without gaining weight.

The amount of food energy required to sustain a given weight is again a function of sex, age, weight, height, and Activity Level. I have programmed still another weight control formula (this one is called the weight maintenance equation); the results of the computer printout are the Weight Maintenance Calorie Tables that follow. These tables make it possible to quickly determine the number of calories per day needed to maintain your present weight, your ideal weight, or any weight.

How to Use the Weight Maintenance Calorie Tables

To use the Weight Maintenance Calorie Tables, you should first determine your Activity Level from the table on page 14. Then find the page number for your personal Weight Maintenance Calorie Table from the Index on page 129.

On examination, it can be seen that the Weight Maintenance Calorie Tables are much simpler in design than the Weight Loss Calorie Tables. To find the number of calories per day needed to sustain a given weight, first locate that weight in the left-hand column and then proceed horizontally to the right until the column headed by the proper Activity Level is intersected. The number at the intersection is the maintenance calories needed per day. For example, again consider the 32-year-old female first described on page 36. She was 5'4" and her Activity Level was 2; therefore, her Weight Maintenance Calorie Table is on page 139. At the start of her reducing diet she was 140 pounds. From page 139, we find that the quantity of food she was consuming before the start of her diet must have been equal to 2413 calories per day. Now, after losing fifteen pounds she weighs 125 pounds, and the same Weight Maintenance Calorie Table shows that, in order to maintain her new weight, she must restrict her intake in the future to 2246 calories.

Maintenance Caloric Needs

Two interesting points are revealed by the preceding numerical exercise. First, maintenance caloric needs decrease as weight is lost. This fact is inherently accounted for in the weight change equations upon which this book is based. Therefore, on a weight loss diet, the difference between the calories needed to sustain a given weight and the diet calorie intake also decreases as weight is lost. Since it is this difference which causes weight loss, it follows that the rate at which weight is lost must also decrease as weight is lost (or as the time on the diet increases). The second observation is that once weight is lost, and the reducing diet terminated, to remain at the lower weight one must eat less than before the start of the diet. The fact is that less food is required to sustain the lower body weight.

The Weight Maintenance Calorie Tables are another new weight control tool. In the past, to determine the number of calories needed to maintain a given weight, one had either to settle for the very crude estimates

Weight Maintenance Calorie Tables 129

available or do some research and lengthy calculations to find a more personal maintenance calorie value. Now, however, for the first time, weight maintenance caloric values are available in the easy-to-use tables that follow.

WEIGHT MAINTENANCE CALORIE TABLE INDEX

SEX	HEIGHT	AGE	PAGE NO.
MALE	5′ 0″—5′ 5″	18–35	130
		36–55	131
		56–75	132
MALE	5′ 6″—5′ 11″	18–35	133
		36–55	134
		56–75	135
MALE	6′ 0″—6′ 6″	18–35	136
		36–55	137
		56–75	138
FEMALE	4′ 11″—5′ 5″	18–35	139
		36–55	140
		56–75	141
FEMALE	5′ 6″—6′ 0″	18–35	142
		36–55	143
		56–75	144

WEIGHT MAINTENANCE CALORIE TABLE

Sex: Male Height: 5' 0"—5' 5"
Age: 18–35 Yrs.

WEIGHT LBS.	ACTIVITY			
	LEVEL 1	LEVEL 2	LEVEL 3	LEVEL 4
100	1922	2080	2327	2797
105	1976	2142	2402	2895
110	2030	2203	2475	2992
115	2082	2264	2548	3088
120	2134	2323	2620	3184
125	2185	2383	2691	3279
130	2236	2441	2762	3373
135	2285	2499	2832	3467
140	2335	2556	2902	3560
150	2432	2669	3040	3745
160	2527	2780	3175	3927
170	2621	2890	3309	4108
180	2713	2997	3442	4288
190	2804	3104	3573	4466
200	2893	3209	3703	4643
210	2981	3313	3832	4819
220	3069	3416	3960	4994
230	3155	3518	4086	5167
240	3240	3619	4212	5340
250	3324	3719	4337	5512
260	3407	3818	4460	5682

Values in table: calories per day.

WEIGHT MAINTENANCE CALORIE TABLE

Sex: Male Height: 5' 0"—5' 5"
Age: 36–55 Yrs.

WEIGHT LBS.	ACTIVITY			
	LEVEL 0	LEVEL 1	LEVEL 2	LEVEL 3
100	1771	1841	1999	2246
105	1820	1893	2059	2318
110	1868	1945	2119	2390
115	1915	1996	2177	2461
120	1962	2046	2236	2532
125	2008	2096	2293	2602
130	2054	2145	2350	2671
135	2098	2193	2406	2740
140	2143	2241	2462	2808
150	2230	2335	2572	2943
160	2316	2428	2681	3076
170	2400	2519	2788	3207
180	2483	2609	2893	3338
190	2564	2697	2997	3466
200	2644	2784	3100	3594
210	2723	2870	3202	3720
220	2801	2955	3302	3846
230	2878	3039	3402	3970
240	2954	3122	3501	4094
250	3029	3204	3599	4216
260	3103	3285	3696	4338

Values in table: calories per day.

WEIGHT MAINTENANCE CALORIE TABLE

Sex: Male Height: 5′ 0″—5′ 5″
Age: 56–75 Yrs.

WEIGHT LBS.	ACTIVITY			
	LEVEL 0	LEVEL 1	LEVEL 2	LEVEL 3
100	1682	1752	1910	2157
105	1729	1803	1969	2228
110	1776	1853	2026	2298
115	1821	1902	2083	2368
120	1866	1950	2140	2436
125	1911	1998	2196	2504
130	1955	2046	2251	2572
135	1998	2092	2306	2639
140	2041	2139	2360	2706
150	2125	2230	2467	2838
160	2208	2320	2573	2968
170	2289	2408	2677	3097
180	2369	2495	2779	3224
190	2448	2581	2881	3350
200	2525	2665	2981	3475
210	2602	2749	3080	3599
220	2677	2831	3179	3722
230	2752	2913	3276	3844
240	2825	2993	3373	3965
250	2898	3073	3468	4086
260	2970	3152	3563	4205

Values in table: calories per day.

WEIGHT MAINTENANCE CALORIE TABLE

Sex: Male Height: 5' 6"—5' 11"
Age: 18–35 Yrs.

WEIGHT LBS.	ACTIVITY			
	LEVEL 1	LEVEL 2	LEVEL 3	LEVEL 4
120	2245	2434	2731	3295
125	2298	2495	2804	3392
130	2350	2556	2877	3488
135	2402	2615	2949	3583
140	2453	2674	3020	3678
145	2504	2733	3091	3773
150	2554	2791	3161	3866
155	2604	2848	3231	3960
160	2653	2905	3301	4053
170	2750	3018	3438	4237
180	2845	3129	3574	4420
190	2939	3239	3708	4601
200	3031	3347	3841	4781
210	3122	3454	3973	4960
220	3212	3560	4103	5137
230	3301	3664	4232	5313
240	3389	3768	4361	5489
250	3476	3871	4488	5663
260	3562	3972	4615	5837
270	3647	4073	4740	6009
280	3731	4173	4865	6181

Values in table: calories per day.

WEIGHT MAINTENANCE CALORIE TABLE

Sex: Male Height: 5' 6"—5' 11"
Age: 36–55 Yrs.

WEIGHT LBS.	ACTIVITY			
	LEVEL 0	LEVEL 1	LEVEL 2	LEVEL 3
120	2031	2115	2304	2601
125	2078	2166	2363	2672
130	2125	2216	2421	2742
135	2171	2265	2479	2812
140	2216	2314	2536	2881
145	2261	2363	2592	2950
150	2306	2411	2648	3018
155	2350	2459	2703	3086
160	2394	2506	2759	3154
170	2480	2599	2867	3287
180	2564	2690	2975	3419
190	2648	2781	3081	3550
200	2729	2869	3185	3679
210	2810	2957	3289	3808
220	2890	3044	3391	3935
230	2968	3129	3493	4061
240	3046	3214	3593	4186
250	3123	3298	3693	4310
260	3199	3381	3792	4434
270	3274	3463	3890	4557
280	3349	3545	3987	4679

Values in table: calories per day.

WEIGHT MAINTENANCE CALORIE TABLE

Sex: Male Height: 5′ 6″—5′ 11″
Age: 56–75 Yrs.

WEIGHT LBS.	ACTIVITY			
	LEVEL 0	LEVEL 1	LEVEL 2	LEVEL 3
120	1927	2011	2201	2497
125	1973	2060	2258	2567
130	2018	2109	2314	2635
135	2062	2157	2370	2704
140	2106	2204	2425	2771
145	2150	2251	2480	2838
150	2192	2297	2534	2905
155	2235	2343	2588	2971
160	2277	2389	2642	3037
170	2360	2479	2748	3168
180	2442	2568	2852	3297
190	2522	2655	2955	3425
200	2601	2741	3057	3551
210	2679	2826	3158	3677
220	2756	2910	3258	3801
230	2832	2993	3357	3925
240	2907	3075	3455	4047
250	2982	3157	3552	4169
260	3055	3237	3648	4290
270	3128	3317	3744	4411
280	3201	3397	3839	4531

Values in table: calories per day.

WEIGHT MAINTENANCE CALORIE TABLE

Sex: Male Height: 6' 0"—6' 6"
Age: 18–35 Yrs.

WEIGHT LBS.	ACTIVITY			
	LEVEL 1	LEVEL 2	LEVEL 3	LEVEL 4
140	2551	2772	3118	3776
145	2603	2832	3191	3872
150	2655	2892	3262	3967
155	2706	2951	3334	4062
160	2756	3009	3404	4156
165	2806	3067	3475	4250
170	2856	3125	3545	4344
175	2905	3182	3614	4436
180	2954	3238	3683	4529
190	3050	3350	3820	4713
200	3145	3461	3955	4895
210	3239	3570	4089	5076
220	3331	3678	4222	5256
230	3422	3785	4353	5434
240	3512	3891	4484	5612
250	3601	3996	4613	5788
260	3689	4100	4742	5964
270	3776	4203	4870	6139
280	3863	4305	4997	6313
290	3948	4406	5123	6486
300	4033	4507	5248	6658

Values in table: calories per day.

WEIGHT MAINTENANCE CALORIE TABLE

Sex: Male Height: 6' 0"—6' 6"
Age: 36–55 Yrs.

WEIGHT LBS.	ACTIVITY			
	LEVEL 0	LEVEL 1	LEVEL 2	LEVEL 3
140	2355	2453	2674	3020
145	2402	2504	2733	3091
150	2449	2554	2791	3161
155	2495	2604	2848	3231
160	2541	2653	2905	3301
165	2586	2701	2962	3370
170	2631	2750	3018	3438
175	2675	2797	3074	3506
180	2719	2845	3129	3574
190	2806	2939	3239	3708
200	2891	3031	3347	3841
210	2975	3122	3454	3973
220	3058	3212	3560	4103
230	3140	3301	3664	4232
240	3221	3389	3768	4361
250	3301	3476	3871	4488
260	3380	3562	3972	4615
270	3458	3647	4073	4740
280	3535	3731	4173	4865
290	3612	3815	4273	4989
300	3687	3897	4371	5112

Values in table: calories per day.

WEIGHT MAINTENANCE CALORIE TABLE

Sex: Male Height: 6' 0"—6' 6"
Age: 56–75 Yrs.

WEIGHT LBS.	ACTIVITY			
	LEVEL 0	LEVEL 1	LEVEL 2	LEVEL 3
140	2237	2335	2556	2902
145	2282	2384	2613	2971
150	2327	2432	2669	3040
155	2371	2480	2725	3108
160	2415	2527	2780	3175
165	2459	2574	2835	3243
170	2502	2621	2890	3309
175	2545	2667	2944	3376
180	2587	2713	2997	3442
190	2671	2804	3104	3573
200	2753	2893	3209	3703
210	2834	2981	3313	3832
220	2915	3069	3416	3960
230	2994	3155	3518	4086
240	3072	3240	3619	4212
250	3149	3324	3719	4337
260	3225	3407	3818	4460
270	3301	3490	3917	4584
280	3376	3572	4014	4706
290	3450	3653	4111	4828
300	3524	3734	4208	4949

Values in table: calories per day.

WEIGHT MAINTENANCE CALORIE TABLE

Sex: Female Height: 4' 11"—5' 5"
Age: 18–35 Yrs.

WEIGHT LBS.	ACTIVITY			
	LEVEL 0	LEVEL 1	LEVEL 2	LEVEL 3
100	1728	1798	1956	2203
105	1776	1850	2016	2275
110	1824	1901	2074	2346
115	1870	1951	2132	2416
120	1916	2000	2190	2486
125	1961	2049	2246	2555
130	2006	2097	2302	2624
135	2050	2145	2358	2691
140	2094	2192	2413	2759
145	2137	2239	2468	2826
150	2180	2285	2522	2892
160	2264	2376	2629	3024
170	2347	2466	2734	3154
180	2428	2554	2838	3283
190	2508	2641	2941	3411
200	2587	2727	3043	3537
210	2665	2812	3143	3662
220	2741	2895	3243	3786
230	2817	2978	3342	3910
240	2892	3060	3439	4032
250	2966	3141	3536	4154

Values in table: calories per day.

WEIGHT MAINTENANCE CALORIE TABLE

Sex: Female   Height: 4' 11"—5' 5"
Age: 36–55 Yrs.

WEIGHT LBS.	ACTIVITY			
	LEVEL 0	LEVEL 1	LEVEL 2	LEVEL 3
100	1682	1752	1910	2157
105	1729	1803	1969	2228
110	1776	1853	2026	2298
115	1821	1902	2083	2368
120	1866	1950	2140	2436
125	1911	1998	2196	2504
130	1955	2046	2251	2572
135	1998	2092	2306	2639
140	2041	2139	2360	2706
145	2083	2185	2414	2772
150	2125	2230	2467	2838
160	2208	2320	2573	2968
170	2289	2408	2677	3097
180	2369	2495	2779	3224
190	2448	2581	2881	3350
200	2525	2665	2981	3475
210	2602	2749	3080	3599
220	2677	2831	3179	3722
230	2752	2913	3276	3844
240	2825	2993	3373	3965
250	2898	3073	3468	4086

Values in table: calories per day.

WEIGHT MAINTENANCE CALORIE TABLE

Sex: Female Height: 4' 11"—5' 5"
Age: 56–75 Yrs.

WEIGHT LBS.	ACTIVITY			
	LEVEL 0	LEVEL 1	LEVEL 2	LEVEL 3
100	1608	1678	1836	2083
105	1653	1727	1893	2152
110	1698	1775	1949	2221
115	1742	1823	2005	2289
120	1786	1870	2060	2356
125	1829	1916	2114	2423
130	1871	1962	2168	2489
135	1913	2008	2221	2555
140	1955	2053	2274	2620
145	1996	2098	2327	2685
150	2037	2142	2379	2749
160	2117	2229	2482	2877
170	2196	2315	2584	3003
180	2274	2400	2684	3129
190	2350	2483	2783	3252
200	2425	2565	2881	3375
210	2500	2647	2978	3497
220	2573	2727	3075	3618
230	2646	2807	3170	3738
240	2717	2885	3265	3857
250	2789	2964	3359	3976

Values in table: calories per day.

WEIGHT MAINTENANCE CALORIE TABLE

Sex: Female Height: 5' 6"—6' 0"
Age: 18–35 Yrs.

WEIGHT LBS.	ACTIVITY			
	LEVEL 0	LEVEL 1	LEVEL 2	LEVEL 3
100	1820	1890	2048	2295
105	1870	1944	2110	2369
110	1919	1996	2170	2442
115	1968	2048	2230	2514
120	2015	2099	2289	2585
125	2062	2150	2347	2656
130	2109	2200	2405	2726
135	2155	2249	2463	2796
140	2200	2298	2519	2865
145	2245	2346	2575	2934
150	2289	2394	2631	3002
160	2376	2488	2741	3136
170	2462	2581	2850	3270
180	2546	2672	2957	3401
190	2629	2762	3062	3531
200	2710	2850	3166	3660
210	2791	2938	3270	3788
220	2870	3024	3372	3915
230	2948	3109	3473	4041
240	3026	3194	3573	4166
250	3102	3277	3672	4290

Values in table: calories per day.

WEIGHT MAINTENANCE CALORIE TABLE

Sex: Female   Height: 5′ 6″—6′ 0″
Age: 36–55 Yrs.

WEIGHT LBS.	ACTIVITY			
	LEVEL 0	LEVEL 1	LEVEL 2	LEVEL 3
100	1739	1809	1967	2214
105	1787	1861	2027	2286
110	1835	1912	2085	2357
115	1881	1962	2144	2428
120	1927	2011	2201	2497
125	1973	2060	2258	2567
130	2018	2109	2314	2635
135	2062	2157	2370	2704
140	2106	2204	2425	2771
145	2150	2251	2480	2838
150	2192	2297	2534	2905
160	2277	2389	2642	3037
170	2360	2479	2748	3168
180	2442	2568	2852	3297
190	2522	2655	2955	3425
200	2601	2741	3057	3551
210	2679	2826	3158	3677
220	2756	2910	3258	3801
230	2832	2993	3357	3925
240	2907	3075	3455	4047
250	2982	3157	3552	4169

Values in table: calories per day.

WEIGHT MAINTENANCE CALORIE TABLE

Sex: Female Height: 5′ 6″—6′ 0″
Age: 56–75 Yrs.

WEIGHT LBS.	ACTIVITY			
	LEVEL 0	LEVEL 1	LEVEL 2	LEVEL 3
100	1665	1735	1893	2140
105	1711	1785	1951	2210
110	1757	1834	2008	2280
115	1803	1883	2065	2349
120	1847	1931	2121	2417
125	1891	1979	2176	2485
130	1935	2026	2231	2552
135	1978	2072	2286	2619
140	2020	2118	2340	2685
145	2062	2164	2393	2751
150	2104	2209	2446	2817
160	2186	2298	2551	2946
170	2267	2386	2655	3074
180	2346	2472	2757	3201
190	2424	2557	2858	3327
200	2501	2641	2957	3451
210	2577	2724	3056	3575
220	2652	2806	3154	3697
230	2726	2887	3251	3819
240	2800	2968	3347	3940
250	2872	3047	3442	4060

Values in table: calories per day.

9. Weight Maintenance Menu Tables

Why is maintenance more difficult than dieting? Primarily because maintenance requires a life-long commitment: a commitment to a new life-style, whereby you eat balanced meals that are within your caloric allowance.

Obviously, any motivational speech I make at this point is not going to be of much help to you five years from now, when hopefully you will still be in a maintenance mode. So, if you really want to keep off that weight, realize now that you will have to practice a good deal of self-discipline for a long time. Even if you are well-motivated, however, in order to succeed you need additional data and a sound weight maintenance plan.

To this end, I have devised still another set of tables, which I call Weight Maintenance Menu Tables. There are 32 of these tables. All were produced on a digital computer, and all represent a complete meal type. The menu tables are similar to the Weight Loss Diet Tables; that is, no specific recipes are given, and the maintenance tables also carry an alpha-numeric designation such as MB-1 (which in this case refers to *M*aintenance *B*reakfast number *1*).

The tables can be used either to plan personal maintenance menus or merely to obtain an idea of what portion sizes of particular meal types can be eaten.

Additional Notes About Menu Tables

1. Again, use the table headed Beverage and Dessert Type Designation (on page 105) to determine the particular beverages or desserts that correspond to the letters designated in the menu tables.
2. Breakfast tables: One slice of French toast (made with one egg for two slices) may be substituted where pancakes are indicated; ½ cup of grits may be eaten in place of a portion of home-fries.

As a general comment, I might add that many of the foods shown in the tables are included because surveys indicate these are the foods people eat. This does not mean that all the foods presented or the portion sizes shown are necessarily recommended.

Remember, if you are to be successful at weight maintenance you must train yourself to eat within your calorie limit. To do this you have to know how to relate calories to meal portion sizes—this is where the Weight Maintenance Menu Tables will prove most valuable.

WEIGHT MAINTENANCE MENU TABLE INDEX

MEAL	BASIS	TYPE	PAGE NO.
Breakfast	Eggs	MB-1	148
	Cereal	MB-2	150
	Pancakes	MB-3	152
	Eggs and Cereal	MB-4	154
	Pancakes and Eggs	MB-5	156
Lunch	Soup and Sandwich	ML-1	158
	Soup and Sandwich	ML-2	160
	Soup and Sandwich	ML-3	162
	Soup and Sandwich	ML-4	164
	Hamburger	ML-5	166
	Frankfurter	ML-6	168
	Omelet	ML-7	170
Dinner	Pot Roast	MD-1	172
	Roast Beef	MD-2	174
	Steak	MD-3	176
	Liver and Onions	MD-4	178
	Lamb Chops	MD-5	180
	Pork Chops	MD-6	182
	Roast Pork	MD-7	184
	Meat Loaf	MD-8	186
	Beef and Vegetable Stew	MD-9	188
	Roast Chicken	MD-10	190
	Fried Chicken	MD-11	192
	Chicken with Vegetables	MD-12	194
	Roast Duck	MD-13	196
	Broiled Fish	MD-14	198
	Fried Fish	MD-15	200
	Seafood Gumbo	MD-16	202
	Lobster	MD-17	204
	Broiled Shrimp	MD-18	206
	Macaroni Casserole	MD-19	208
	Spaghetti and Meat Balls	MD-20	210

WEIGHT MAINTENANCE MENU TABLE

Meal: Breakfast   Type: MB-1

Content: Juice or Fresh Fruit
Eggs, any Style
Bacon or Equivalent
Home-Fries or Equivalent
Toast, Beverage

Calorie Total	Eggs	Juice Oz.	Toast Slices	Bacon Strips	Home Fries	Beverage Type
240	1	4	*	0	0	A
260	1	4	1	0	0	A
300	1	4	1	0	0	B
350	1	4	1	2	0	A
390	1	4	1	2	0	B
440	1	4	2	2	0	A
480	1	4	2	2	0	B
550	1	4	2	2	1	A
590	1	4	2	2	1	B
660	1	6	2	2	1	2-B
380	2	4	1	0	0	A
420	2	4	1	0	0	B
470	2	4	2	0	0	A
510	2	4	2	0	0	B
560	2	4	2	2	0	A
600	2	4	2	2	0	B
670	2	4	2	2	1	A
710	2	4	2	2	1	B
780	2	6	2	2	1	2-B
910	2	6	3	3	1	2-B

Toast is assumed to be spread with ½ pat of butter or margarine. If toast is designated * (plain), use no butter. A portion of home-fries is assumed to be approximately 10 pieces (2 × ½ × ½ inch).

WEIGHT MAINTENANCE MENU TABLE

Meal: Breakfast   Type: MB-1 (Con't)

Calorie Total	Eggs	Juice Oz.	Toast Slices	Bacon Strips	Home Fries	Beverage Type
580	3	4	2	0	0	A
620	3	4	2	0	0	B
670	3	4	2	2	0	A
710	3	4	2	2	0	B
780	3	4	2	2	1	A
820	3	4	2	2	1	B
870	3	6	3	2	0	2-B
960	3	6	3	4	0	2-B
980	3	6	3	2	1	2-B
1070	3	6	3	4	1	2-B

Toast is assumed to be spread with ½ pat of butter or margarine. A portion of home-fries is assumed to be approximately 10 pieces (2 × ½ × ½ inch).

Note: This table is included for completeness. The consumption of three eggs at one meal is definitely not advisable, particularly for men and post-menopausal women, because of the high amount of cholesterol and saturated fat contained in eggs.

WEIGHT MAINTENANCE MENU TABLE

Meal: Breakfast Type: MB-2

Content: Juice
Hot or Cold Cereal
Whole Milk, Sugar
Fresh Fruit for Cereal
Beverage

Calorie Total	Juice Oz.	Cereal Cups	Milk Oz.	Sugar Tbsp.	Fruit Cups	Beverage Type
250	4	1	5	0	0	A
270	4	1	5	1	0	A
290	4	1	5	0	0	B
310	4	1	5	1	0	B
320	4	1	5	0	1/2	A
340	4	1	5	1	1/2	A
360	4	1	5	0	1/2	B
380	4	1	5	1	1/2	B
280	6	1	5	0	0	A
300	6	1	5	1	0	A
320	6	1	5	0	0	B
340	6	1	5	1	0	B
350	6	1	5	0	1/2	A
370	6	1	5	1	1/2	A
390	6	1	5	0	1/2	B
410	6	1	5	1	1/2	B

Try skim milk in place of whole milk. Avoid the butter fat and deduct 40 calories per 5 ounces of milk from the calorie totals listed.

WEIGHT MAINTENANCE MENU TABLE

Meal: Breakfast   Type: MB-2 (Con't)

Calorie Total	Juice Oz.	Cereal Cups	Milk Oz.	Sugar Tbsp.	Fruit Cups	Beverage Type
430	4	2	10	0	0	A
450	4	2	10	1	0	A
470	4	2	10	0	0	B
490	4	2	10	1	0	B
570	4	2	10	0	1	A
590	4	2	10	1	1	A
610	4	2	10	0	1	B
630	4	2	10	1	1	B
450	6	2	10	0	0	A
480	6	2	10	1	0	A
500	6	2	10	0	0	B
520	6	2	10	1	0	B
600	6	2	10	0	1	A
620	6	2	10	1	1	A
640	6	2	10	0	1	B
660	6	2	10	1	1	B

Try skim milk in place of whole milk. Avoid the butter fat and deduct 40 calories per 5 ounces of milk from the calorie totals listed.

WEIGHT MAINTENANCE MENU TABLE

Meal: Breakfast   Type MB-3

Content: Juice or Fresh Fruit
Pancakes or Waffles
Butter, Syrup
Bacon or Equivalent
Beverage

Calorie Total	Juice Oz.	Pancakes	Butter Pats	Syrup Tbsp.	Bacon Strips	Beverage Type
180	4	1	0	0	0	A
220	4	1	0	0	0	B
290	4	1	1/2	1½	0	A
330	4	1	1/2	1½	0	B
340	4	1	1/2	1½	1	A
420	4	1	1/2	1½	2	B
450	6	1	1/2	1½	2	B
480	6	1	1/2	2	2	B
290	4	2	0	0	0	A
380	4	2	1	0	0	B
460	4	2	1	2	0	A
560	4	2	1	3	0	B
610	4	2	1	3	2	A
690	4	2	1	3	2	2-B
720	6	2	1	3	2	2-B
780	6	2	1	4	2	2-B

Pancakes are assumed to be a maximum of 5½ inches in diameter.

WEIGHT MAINTENANCE MENU TABLE

Meal: Breakfast   Type: MB-3 (Con't)

Calorie Total	Juice Oz.	Pan-cakes	Butter Pats	Syrup Tbsp.	Bacon Strips	Beverage Type
450	4	3	1	0	0	A
610	4	3	1	2	0	B
630	4	3	1	3	0	A
780	4	3	1½	4½	0	B
830	4	3	1½	4½	2	A
910	4	3	1½	4½	2	2-B
940	6	3	1½	4½	3	2-B
1060	6	3	1½	5	4	2-B
560	4	4	1	0	0	A
720	4	4	1	2	0	B
800	4	4	1	4	0	A
1010	4	4	2	6	0	B
1060	4	4	2	6	2	A
1140	4	4	2	6	2	2-B
1260	6	4	2	6	4	2-B
1360	6	4	2	7	5	2-B

Pancakes are assumed to be a maximum of 5½ inches in diameter.

WEIGHT MAINTENANCE MENU TABLE

Meal: Breakfast   Type: MB-4

Content: Juice or Fresh Fruit
Eggs, Any Style
Hot or Cold Cereal
Bacon or Equivalent
Toast, Beverage

Calorie Total	Juice Oz.	Eggs	Cereal Cups	Bacon Strips	Toast Slices	Beverage Type
360	4	1	1	0	0	A
420	4	1	1	0	*	A
450	4	1	1	0	1	A
490	4	1	1	0	1	B
500	4	1	1	1	1	A
540	4	1	1	1	1	B
590	4	1	1	1	2	A
630	4	1	1	1	2	B
670	6	1	1	2	2	A
710	6	1	1	2	2	B
470	4	2	1	0	0	A
560	4	2	1	0	1	A
600	4	2	1	0	1	B
650	4	2	1	0	2	A
690	4	2	1	0	2	B
740	4	2	1	2	2	A
780	4	2	1	2	2	B
780	6	2	1	2	2	A
820	6	2	1	2	2	B
950	6	2	1	2	3	2-B

Toast is assumed to be spread with ½ pat of butter or margarine. If toast is designated * (plain), use no butter. Cereal is assumed to contain a maximum of 5 ounces of whole milk (skim milk is preferable).

WEIGHT MAINTENANCE MENU TABLE

Meal: Breakfast   Type: MB-4 (Con't)

Calorie Total	Juice Oz.	Eggs	Cereal Cups	Bacon Strips	Toast Slices	Beverage Type
670	4	3	1	0	1	A
760	4	3	1	0	2	A
800	4	3	1	0	2	B
850	4	3	1	2	2	A
890	4	3	1	2	2	B
920	6	3	1	2	2	B
960	6	3	1	2	2	2-B
1050	6	3	1	4	2	2-B
1140	6	3	1	4	3	2-B
1230	6	3	1	4	4	2-B

Toast is assumed to be spread with ½ pat of butter or margarine. Cereal is assumed to contain a maximum of 5 ounces of whole milk (skim milk is preferable).

Note: This table is included for completeness. The consumption of three eggs at one meal is definitely not advisable, particularly for men and post-menopausal women, because of the high amount of cholesterol and saturated fat contained in eggs.

WEIGHT MAINTENANCE MENU TABLE

Meal: Breakfast   Type: MB-5

Content: Juice or Fresh Fruit
Pancakes or Waffles
Eggs, any Style
Butter, Syrup
Beverage

Calorie Total	Juice Oz.	Pan-cakes	Eggs	Butter Pats	Syrup Tbsp.	Beverage Type
290	4	1	1	0	0	A
350	4	1	1	1/2	0	B
400	4	1	1	1/2	1½	A
440	4	1	1	1/2	1½	B
540	6	1	1	1/2	2	2-B
400	4	1	2	0	0	A
460	4	1	2	1/2	0	B
510	4	1	2	1/2	1½	A
550	4	1	2	1/2	1½	B
650	6	1	2	1/2	2	2-B
400	4	2	1	0	0	A
490	4	2	1	1	0	B
630	4	2	1	1	3	A
670	4	2	1	1	3	B
800	6	2	1	1	4	2-B

Pancakes are assumed to be a maximum of 5½ inches in diameter.

WEIGHT MAINTENANCE MENU TABLE

Meal: Breakfast   Type: MB-5 (Con't)

Calorie Total	Juice Oz.	Pan-cakes	Eggs	Butter Pats	Syrup Tbsp.	Beverage Type
510	4	2	2	0	0	A
600	4	2	2	1	0	B
740	4	2	2	1	3	A
820	4	2	2	1	3	2-B
910	6	2	2	1	4	2-B
510	4	3	1	0	0	A
600	4	3	1	1	0	B
850	4	3	1	1½	4½	A
930	4	3	1	1½	4½	2-B
990	6	3	1	1½	5	2-B
670	4	4	1	1	0	A
760	4	4	1	2	0	B
1080	4	4	1	2	6	A
1160	4	4	1	2	6	2-B
1250	6	4	1	2	7	2-B

Pancakes are assumed to be a maximum of 5½ inches in diameter.

WEIGHT MAINTENANCE MENU TABLE

Meal: Lunch   Type: ML-1

Content: Soup (Water Base) and/or Sandwich (2 oz. Meat or Cheese) Beverage, Dessert

Calorie Total	No. of Sandwiches	Soup Cups	Beverage Type	Dessert Type
470	1	0	A	A
470	1	0	B	None
510	1	0	B	A
560	1	0	C	A
570	1	0	D	None
670	1	0	A	C
710	1	0	B	C
820	1	0	D	C
570	1	1	A	A
570	1	1	B	None
610	1	1	B	A
660	1	1	C	A
670	1	1	D	None
770	1	1	A	C
810	1	1	B	C
920	1	1	D	C

Two ounces of luncheon meat is equivalent to approximately 2 slices of meat (4 × 4 × ⅛ inch). Sandwich is assumed to be spread with a tbsp. of either mayonnaise, butter, or margarine. If catsup or mustard are used, deduct 75 from the calorie totals shown. If no spread is used, deduct 100 calories.

WEIGHT MAINTENANCE MENU TABLE
Meal: Lunch   Type: ML-1 (Con't)

Calorie Total	No. of Sandwiches	Soup Cups	Beverage Type	Dessert Type
890	2	0	A	A
890	2	0	B	None
930	2	0	B	A
980	2	0	C	A
990	2	0	D	None
1090	2	0	A	C
1130	2	0	B	C
1240	2	0	D	C
990	2	1	A	A
990	2	1	B	None
1030	2	1	B	A
1080	2	1	C	A
1090	2	1	D	None
1190	2	1	A	C
1230	2	1	B	C
1340	2	1	D	C

Two ounces of luncheon meat is equivalent to approximately 2 slices of meat (4 × 4 × ⅛ inch). Sandwich is assumed to be spread with a tbsp. of either mayonnaise, butter, or margarine. If catsup or mustard are used, deduct 75 from the calorie totals shown. If no spread is used, deduct 100 calories.

WEIGHT MAINTENANCE MENU TABLE

Meal: Lunch   Type: ML-2

Content: Soup (Milk Base) and/or
Sandwich (2 oz. Meat or Cheese)
Beverage, Dessert

Calorie Total	No. of Sandwiches	Soup Cups	Beverage Type	Dessert Type
470	1	0	A	A
470	1	0	B	None
510	1	0	B	A
560	1	0	C	A
570	1	0	D	None
670	1	0	A	C
710	1	0	B	C
820	1	0	D	C
670	1	1	A	A
670	1	1	B	None
710	1	1	B	A
760	1	1	C	A
770	1	1	D	None
870	1	1	A	C
910	1	1	B	C
1020	1	1	D	C

Two ounces of luncheon meat is equivalent to approximately 2 slices of meat (4 × 4 × ⅛ inch). Sandwich is assumed to be spread with a tbsp. of either mayonnaise, butter, or margarine. If catsup or mustard are used, deduct 75 from the calorie totals shown. If no spread is used, deduct 100 calories.

WEIGHT MAINTENANCE MENU TABLE
Meal: Lunch   Type: ML-2 (Con't)

Calorie Total	No. of Sandwiches	Soup Cups	Beverage Type	Dessert Type
890	2	0	A	A
890	2	0	B	None
930	2	0	B	A
980	2	0	C	A
990	2	0	D	None
1090	2	0	A	C
1130	2	0	B	C
1240	2	0	D	C
1090	2	1	A	A
1090	2	1	B	None
1130	2	1	B	A
1180	2	1	C	A
1190	2	1	D	None
1290	2	1	A	C
1330	2	1	B	C
1440	2	1	D	C

Two ounces of luncheon meat is equivalent to approximately 2 slices of meat (4 × 4 × ⅛ inch). Sandwich is assumed to be spread with a tbsp. of either mayonnaise, butter, or margarine. If catsup or mustard are used, deduct 75 from the calorie totals shown. If no spread is used, deduct 100 calories.

WEIGHT MAINTENANCE MENU TABLE

Meal: Lunch   Type: ML-3

Content: Soup (Water Base) and/or
Sandwich (Salad Type)
Beverage, Dessert

Calorie Total	No. of Sandwiches	Soup Cups	Beverage Type	Dessert Type
390	1	0	A	A
390	1	0	B	None
430	1	0	B	A
480	1	0	C	A
490	1	0	D	None
590	1	0	A	C
630	1	0	B	C
740	1	0	D	C
490	1	1	A	A
490	1	1	B	None
530	1	1	B	A
580	1	1	C	A
590	1	1	D	None
690	1	1	A	C
730	1	1	B	C
840	1	1	D	C

Salad type sandwiches include: egg salad, tuna salad, and bacon, lettuce and tomato. Sandwich is assumed to be spread with a tbsp. of either mayonnaise, butter, or margarine. If no spread is used, deduct 100 from the calorie totals shown.

WEIGHT MAINTENANCE MENU TABLE

Meal: Lunch   Type: ML-3 (Con't)

Calorie Total	No. of Sandwiches	Soup Cups	Beverage Type	Dessert Type
730	2	0	A	A
730	2	0	B	None
770	2	0	B	A
820	2	0	C	A
830	2	0	D	None
930	2	0	A	C
970	2	0	B	C
1080	2	0	D	C
830	2	1	A	A
830	2	1	B	None
870	2	1	B	A
920	2	1	C	A
930	2	1	D	None
1030	2	1	A	C
1070	2	1	B	C
1180	2	1	D	C

Salad type sandwiches include: egg salad, tuna salad, and bacon, lettuce and tomato. Sandwich is assumed to be spread with a tbsp. of either mayonnaise, butter, or margarine. If no spread is used, deduct 100 from the calorie totals shown.

WEIGHT MAINTENANCE MENU TABLE

Meal: Lunch Type: ML-4
Content: Soup (Milk Base) and/or
Sandwich (Salad Type)
Beverage, Dessert

Calorie Total	No. of Sandwiches	Soup Cups	Beverage Type	Dessert Type
390	1	0	A	A
390	1	0	B	None
430	1	0	B	A
480	1	0	C	A
490	1	0	D	None
590	1	0	A	C
630	1	0	B	C
740	1	0	D	C
590	1	1	A	A
590	1	1	B	None
630	1	1	B	A
680	1	1	C	A
690	1	1	D	None
790	1	1	A	C
830	1	1	B	C
940	1	1	D	C

Salad type sandwiches include: egg salad, tuna salad, and bacon, lettuce and tomato. Sandwich is assumed to be spread with a tbsp. of either mayonnaise, butter, or margarine. If no spread is used, deduct 100 from the calorie totals shown.

WEIGHT MAINTENANCE MENU TABLE
Meal: Lunch Type: ML-4 (Con't)

Calorie Total	No. of Sandwiches	Soup Cups	Beverage Type	Dessert Type
730	2	0	A	A
730	2	0	B	None
770	2	0	B	A
820	2	0	C	A
830	2	0	D	None
930	2	0	A	C
970	2	0	B	C
1080	2	0	D	C
930	2	1	A	A
930	2	1	B	None
970	2	1	B	A
1020	2	1	C	A
1030	2	1	D	None
1130	2	1	A	C
1170	2	1	B	C
1280	2	1	D	C

Salad type sandwiches include: egg salad, tuna salad, and bacon, lettuce and tomato. Sandwich is assumed to be spread with a tbsp. of either mayonnaise, butter, or margarine. If no spread is used, deduct 100 from the calorie totals shown.

WEIGHT MAINTENANCE MENU TABLE

Meal: Lunch   Type: ML-5

Content: Hamburger on Roll
French Fried Potatoes
Green Salad with Dressing
Beverage and Dessert

Calorie Total	No. of Hamburgers	French Fries	Salad Dressing Tbsp.	Beverage Type	Dessert Type
370	1	0	0	A	None
460	1	0	0	B	A
520	1	0	0	D	None
780	1	0	2	A	C
820	1	0	2	B	C
920	1	0	2	B	D
930	1	0	2	D	C
1030	1	0	2	D	D
520	1	1	0	A	None
610	1	1	0	B	A
670	1	1	2	D	None
930	1	1	2	A	C
970	1	1	2	B	C
1070	1	1	2	B	D
1080	1	1	2	D	C
1180	1	1	2	D	D

Hamburger is assumed to weigh 3 ounces (4 inch diameter by ⅜ inch thick) after cooking. If mustard or catsup are not used deduct 20 from the calorie totals shown. A portion of French Fries is assumed to be approximately 10 pieces ($2 \times \frac{1}{2} \times \frac{1}{2}$ inch).

WEIGHT MAINTENANCE MENU TABLE

Meal: Lunch   Type: ML-5 (Con't)

Calorie Total	No. of Hamburgers	French Fries	Salad Dressing Tbsp.	Beverage Type	Dessert Type
740	2	0	0	A	None
830	2	0	0	B	A
890	2	0	2	D	None
1150	2	0	2	A	C
1190	2	0	2	B	C
1290	2	0	2	B	D
1300	2	0	2	D	C
1400	2	0	2	D	D
890	2	1	0	A	None
980	2	1	0	B	A
1040	2	1	2	D	None
1300	2	1	2	A	C
1340	2	1	2	B	C
1440	2	1	2	B	D
1450	2	1	2	D	C
1550	2	1	2	D	D

Hamburger is assumed to weigh 3 ounces (4 inch diameter by ⅜ inch thick) after cooking. If mustard or catsup are not used deduct 20 from the calorie totals shown. A portion of French Fries is assumed to be approximately 10 pieces (2 × ½ × ½ inch).

WEIGHT MAINTENANCE MENU TABLE

Meal: Lunch   Type: ML-6
Content: Frankfurter on Roll
French Fried Potatoes
Green Salad with Dressing
Beverage and Dessert

Calorie Total	No. of Franks	French Fries	Salad Dressing Tbsp.	Beverage Type	Dessert Type
300	1	0	0	A	None
390	1	0	0	B	A
450	1	0	0	D	None
710	1	0	2	A	C
750	1	0	2	B	C
850	1	0	2	B	D
860	1	0	2	D	C
960	1	0	2	D	D
450	1	1	0	A	None
540	1	1	0	B	A
600	1	1	0	D	None
860	1	1	2	A	C
900	1	1	2	B	C
1000	1	1	2	B	D
1010	1	1	2	D	C
1110	1	1	2	D	D

Frankfurter is assumed to weigh 2 ounces (8 franks to a one-pound package). If mustard or catsup are not used deduct 20 from the calorie totals shown. A portion of French Fries is assumed to be approximately 10 pieces (2 × ½ × ½ inch).

WEIGHT MAINTENANCE MENU TABLE

Meal: Lunch Type: ML-6 (Con't)

Calorie Total	No. of Franks	French Fries	Salad Dressing Tbsp.	Beverage Type	Dessert Type
600	2	0	0	A	None
690	2	0	0	B	A
750	2	0	0	D	None
1010	2	0	2	A	C
1050	2	0	2	B	C
1150	2	0	2	B	D
1160	2	0	2	D	C
1260	2	0	2	D	D
750	2	1	0	A	None
840	2	1	0	B	A
900	2	1	0	D	None
1160	2	1	2	A	C
1200	2	1	2	B	C
1300	2	1	2	B	D
1310	2	1	2	D	C
1410	2	1	2	D	D

Frankfurter is assumed to weigh 2 ounces (8 franks to a one-pound package). If mustard or catsup are not used deduct 20 from the calorie totals shown. A portion of French Fries is assumed to be approximately 10 pieces ($2 \times \frac{1}{2} \times \frac{1}{2}$ inch).

WEIGHT MAINTENANCE MENU TABLE

Meal: Lunch Type: ML-7
Content: Omelet
French Fried Potatoes
Green Salad with Dressing
Bread, Beverage, and Dessert

Calorie Total	Eggs	French Fries	Salad Dressing Tbsp.	Bread Slices	Beverage Type	Dessert Type
200	1	0	0	0	A	A
330	1	0	0	1	B	A
490	1	0	2	1	B	A
590	1	0	2	1	B	B
640	1	0	2	1	C	B
740	1	1	2	1	B	B
790	1	1	2	1	C	B
890	1	1	2	1	C	C
950	1	1	2	1	D	C
990	1	1	2	1	C	D
1140	1	1	2	2	D	D
350	2	0	0	0	A	A
480	2	0	0	1	B	A
640	2	0	2	1	B	A
740	2	0	2	1	B	B
790	2	0	2	1	C	B
890	2	1	2	1	B	B
940	2	1	2	1	C	B
1040	2	1	2	1	C	C
1190	2	1	2	2	D	C
1230	2	1	2	2	C	D
1290	2	1	2	2	D	D

Omelet types include: western, mushroom, cheese, Spanish, and pepper. A portion of French Fries is assumed to be approximately 10 pieces ($2 \times \frac{1}{2} \times \frac{1}{2}$ inch).

WEIGHT MAINTENANCE MENU TABLE

Meal: Lunch Type: ML-7 (Con't)

Calorie Total	Eggs	French Fries	Salad Dressing Tbsp.	Bread Slices	Beverage Type	Dessert Type
500	3	0	0	0	A	A
630	3	0	0	1	B	A
790	3	0	2	1	B	A
890	3	0	2	1	B	B
940	3	0	2	1	C	B
1130	3	1	2	2	B	B
1180	3	1	2	2	C	B
1280	3	1	2	2	C	C
1340	3	1	2	2	D	C
1380	3	1	2	2	C	D
1440	3	1	2	2	D	D

Omelet types include: western, mushroom, cheese, Spanish, and pepper. A portion of French Fries is assumed to be approximately 10 pieces (2 × ½ × ½ inch).

WEIGHT MAINTENANCE MENU TABLE

Meal: Dinner   Type: MD-1

Content: Pot Roast of Beef
Boiled, Mashed, or Baked Potato
Half-cup Fresh or Cooked Vegetables
Green Salad with Dressing
Bread, Beverage, and Dessert

Calorie Total	Meat Oz.	Potato	Gravy Tbsp.	Salad Dressing Tbsp.	Bread Slices	Beverage Type	Dessert Type
290	4	0	0	0	0	A	None
410	4	0	0	1	0	B	None
530	4	1	0	1	0	B	None
790	4	1	1	2	1	B	A
880	4	1	2	2	1	C	A
940	4	1	2	2	1	D	A
940	4	1	2	2	1	B	B
1030	4	1	2	2	1	B	C
1130	4	1	2	2	1	B	D
1140	4	1	2	2	1	D	C
1330	4	1	2	2	2	D	D
530	8	0	0	0	0	A	None
650	8	0	0	1	0	B	None
770	8	1	0	1	0	B	None

Tabulation assumes ½ cup of vegetables and an unlimited amount of green salad are served with each portion. Where indicated, potato is medium size and prepared with ½ pat of butter, and bread is spread with ½ pat of butter or margarine. As a guide to judging portion size, a slice of meat 4 × 4 × ⅛ inch weighs approximately 2 ounces.

WEIGHT MAINTENANCE MENU TABLE

Meal: Dinner   Type: MD-1 (Con't)

Calorie Total	Meat Oz.	Potato	Gravy Tbsp.	Salad Dressing Tbsp.	Bread Slices	Beverage Type	Dessert Type
1070	8	1	2	2	1	B	A
1160	8	1	3	2	1	C	A
1220	8	1	3	2	1	D	A
1220	8	1	3	2	1	B	B
1310	8	1	3	2	1	B	C
1410	8	1	3	2	1	B	D
1420	8	1	3	2	1	D	C
1610	8	1	3	2	2	D	D
770	12	0	0	0	0	A	None
890	12	0	0	1	0	B	None
1010	12	1	0	1	0	B	None
1350	12	1	3	2	1	B	A
1480	12	1	5	2	1	C	A
1540	12	1	5	2	1	D	A
1540	12	1	5	2	1	B	B
1630	12	1	5	2	1	B	C
1730	12	1	5	2	1	B	D
1740	12	1	5	2	1	D	C
1930	12	1	5	2	2	D	D

Tabulation assumes ½ cup of vegetables and an unlimited amount of green salad are served with each portion. Where indicated, potato is medium size and prepared with ½ pat of butter, and bread is spread with ½ pat of butter or margarine. As a guide to judging portion size, a slice of meat 4 × 4 × ⅛ inch weighs approximately 2 ounces.

WEIGHT MAINTENANCE MENU TABLE

Meal: Dinner   Type: MD-2

Content: Oven Roast of Beef
Boiled, Mashed, or Baked Potato
Half-cup Fresh or Cooked Vegetables
Green Salad with Dressing
Bread, Beverage, and Dessert

Calorie Total	Meat Oz.	Potato	Gravy Tbsp.	Salad Dressing Tbsp.	Bread Slices	Beverage Type	Dessert Type
370	4	0	0	0	0	A	None
490	4	0	0	1	0	B	None
610	4	1	0	1	0	B	None
870	4	1	1	2	1	B	A
960	4	1	2	2	1	C	A
1020	4	1	2	2	1	D	A
1020	4	1	2	2	1	B	B
1110	4	1	2	2	1	B	C
1210	4	1	2	2	1	B	D
1220	4	1	2	2	1	D	C
1320	4	1	2	2	2	D	D
690	8	0	0	0	0	A	None
810	8	0	0	1	0	B	None
930	8	1	0	1	0	B	None

Tabulation assumes ½ cup of vegetables and an unlimited amount of green salad are served with each portion. Where indicated, potato is medium size and prepared with ½ pat of butter, and bread is spread with ½ pat of butter or margarine. As a guide to judging portion size, a slice of meat 4 × 4 × ⅛ inch weighs approximately 2 ounces.

WEIGHT MAINTENANCE MENU TABLE

Meal: Dinner   Type: MD-2 (Con't)

Calorie Total	Meat Oz.	Potato	Gravy Tbsp.	Salad Dressing Tbsp.	Bread Slices	Beverage Type	Dessert Type
1230	8	1	2	2	1	B	A
1320	8	1	3	2	1	C	A
1380	8	1	3	2	1	D	A
1380	8	1	3	2	1	B	B
1470	8	1	3	2	1	B	C
1570	8	1	3	2	1	B	D
1580	8	1	3	2	1	D	C
1770	8	1	3	2	2	D	D
1010	12	0	0	0	0	A	None
1130	12	0	0	1	0	B	None
1250	12	1	0	1	0	B	None
1590	12	1	3	2	1	B	A
1720	12	1	5	2	1	C	A
1780	12	1	5	2	1	D	A
1780	12	1	5	2	1	B	B
1870	12	1	5	2	1	B	C
1970	12	1	5	2	1	B	D
1980	12	1	5	2	1	D	C
2170	12	1	5	2	2	D	D

Tabulation assumes ½ cup of vegetables and an unlimited amount of green salad are served with each portion. Where indicated, potato is medium size and prepared with ½ pat of butter, and bread is spread with ½ pat of butter or margarine. As a guide to judging portion size, a slice of meat 4 × 4 × ⅛ inch weighs approximately 2 ounces.

WEIGHT MAINTENANCE MENU TABLE

Meal: Dinner   Type: MD-3

Content: Broiled Beef Steak
Boiled, Mashed, or Baked Potato
Half-cup Fresh or Cooked Vegetables
Green Salad with Dressing
Bread, Beverage, and Dessert

Calorie Total	Meat Oz.	Potato	Salad Dressing Tbsp.	Bread Slices	Beverage Type	Dessert Type
330	4	0	0	0	A	None
450	4	0	1	0	B	None
570	4	1	1	0	B	None
790	4	1	2	1	B	A
840	4	1	2	1	C	A
900	4	1	2	1	D	A
900	4	1	2	1	B	B
990	4	1	2	1	B	C
1090	4	1	2	1	B	D
1100	4	1	2	1	D	C
1290	4	1	2	2	D	D
610	8	0	0	0	A	None
730	8	0	1	0	B	None
850	8	1	1	0	B	None

Tabulation assumes ½ cup of vegetables and an unlimited amount of green salad are served with each portion. Where indicated, potato is medium size and prepared with ½ pat of butter, and bread is spread with ½ pat of butter or margarine. As a guide to judging portion size, a slice of meat 4 × 4 × ⅛ inch weighs approximately 2 ounces.

WEIGHT MAINTENANCE MENU TABLE

Meal: Dinner   Type: MD-3 (Con't)

Calorie Total	Meat Oz.	Potato	Salad Dressing Tbsp.	Bread Slices	Beverage Type	Dessert Type
1070	8	1	2	1	B	A
1120	8	1	2	1	C	A
1180	8	1	2	1	D	A
1180	8	1	2	1	B	B
1270	8	1	2	1	B	C
1370	8	1	2	1	B	D
1380	8	1	2	1	D	C
1570	8	1	2	2	D	D
890	12	0	0	0	A	None
1010	12	0	1	0	B	None
1130	12	1	1	0	B	None
1350	12	1	2	1	B	A
1400	12	1	2	1	C	A
1460	12	1	2	1	D	A
1460	12	1	2	1	B	B
1550	12	1	2	1	B	C
1650	12	1	2	1	B	D
1660	12	1	2	1	D	C
1850	12	1	2	2	D	D

Tabulation assumes ½ cup of vegetables and an unlimited amount of green salad are served with each portion. Where indicated, potato is medium size and prepared with ½ pat of butter, and bread is spread with ½ pat of butter or margarine. As a guide to judging portion size, a slice of meat 4 × 4 × ⅛ inch weighs approximately 2 ounces.

WEIGHT MAINTENANCE MENU TABLE

Meal: Dinner   Type: MD-4

Content: Fried Liver and Onions
          Boiled, Mashed, or Baked
            Potato
          Half-cup Fresh or Cooked
            Vegetables
          Green Salad with Dressing
          Bread, Beverage, and Dessert

Calorie Total	Meat Oz.	Potato	Salad Dressing Tbsp.	Bread Slices	Beverage Type	Dessert Type
310	4	0	0	0	A	None
430	4	0	1	0	B	None
550	4	1	1	0	B	None
770	4	1	2	1	B	A
820	4	1	2	1	C	A
880	4	1	2	1	D	A
880	4	1	2	1	B	B
970	4	1	2	1	B	C
1070	4	1	2	1	B	D
1080	4	1	2	1	D	C
1270	4	1	2	2	D	D
570	8	0	0	0	A	None
690	8	0	1	0	B	None
810	8	1	1	0	B	None

Tabulation assumes ½ cup of vegetables and an unlimited amount of green salad are served with each portion. Where indicated, potato is medium size and prepared with ½ pat of butter, and bread is spread with ½ pat of butter or margarine. As a guide to judging portion size, a slice of meat $4 \times 4 \times ⅛$ inch weighs approximately 2 ounces.

WEIGHT MAINTENANCE MENU TABLE

Meal: Dinner   Type: MD-4 (Con't)

Calorie Total	Meat Oz.	Potato	Salad Dressing Tbsp.	Bread Slices	Beverage Type	Dessert Type
1030	8	1	2	1	B	A
1080	8	1	2	1	C	A
1140	8	1	2	1	D	A
1140	8	1	2	1	B	B
1230	8	1	2	1	B	C
1330	8	1	2	1	B	D
1340	8	1	2	1	D	C
1530	8	1	2	2	D	D
830	12	0	0	0	A	None
950	12	0	1	0	B	None
1070	12	1	1	0	B	None
1290	12	1	2	1	B	A
1340	12	1	2	1	C	A
1400	12	1	2	1	D	A
1400	12	1	2	1	B	B
1490	12	1	2	1	B	C
1590	12	1	2	1	B	D
1600	12	1	2	1	D	C
1790	12	1	2	2	D	D

Tabulation assumes ½ cup of vegetables and an unlimited amount of green salad are served with each portion. Where indicated, potato is medium size and prepared with ½ pat of butter, and bread is spread with ½ pat of butter or margarine. As a guide to judging portion size, a slice of meat 4 × 4 × ⅛ inch weighs approximately 2 ounces.

WEIGHT MAINTENANCE MENU TABLE

Meal: Dinner Type: MD-5

Content: Rib Lamb Chops
Boiled, Mashed, or Baked Potato
Half-cup Fresh or Cooked Vegetables
Green Salad with Dressing
Bread, Beverage, and Dessert

Calorie Total	No. of Chops	Potato	Salad Dressing Tbsp.	Bread Slices	Beverage Type	Dessert Type
240	1	0	0	0	A	None
360	1	0	1	0	B	None
480	1	1	1	0	B	None
700	1	1	2	1	B	A
750	1	1	2	1	C	A
810	1	1	2	1	D	A
810	1	1	2	1	B	B
900	1	1	2	1	B	C
1000	1	1	2	1	B	D
1010	1	1	2	1	D	C
1200	1	1	2	2	D	D
430	2	0	0	0	A	None
550	2	0	1	0	B	None
670	2	1	1	0	B	None

Tabulation assumes ½ cup of vegetables and an unlimited amount of green salad are served with each portion. Where indicated, potato is medium size and prepared with ½ pat of butter, and bread is spread with ½ pat of butter or margarine. Chops are assumed to weigh approximately ¼ pound each, including bone.

WEIGHT MAINTENANCE MENU TABLE

Meal: Dinner   Type: MD-5 (Con't)

Calorie Total	No. of Chops	Potato	Salad Dressing Tbsp.	Bread Slices	Beverage Type	Dessert Type
890	2	1	2	1	B	A
940	2	1	2	1	C	A
1000	2	1	2	1	D	A
1000	2	1	2	1	B	B
1090	2	1	2	1	B	C
1190	2	1	2	1	B	D
1200	2	1	2	1	D	C
1390	2	1	2	2	D	D
810	4	0	0	0	A	None
930	4	0	1	0	B	None
1050	4	1	1	0	B	None
1270	4	1	2	1	B	A
1320	4	1	2	1	C	A
1380	4	1	2	1	D	A
1380	4	1	2	1	B	B
1470	4	1	2	1	B	C
1570	4	1	2	1	B	D
1580	4	1	2	1	D	C
1770	4	1	2	2	D	D

Tabulation assumes ½ cup of vegetables and an unlimited amount of green salad are served with each portion. Where indicated, potato is medium size and prepared with ½ pat of butter, and bread is spread with ½ pat of butter or margarine. Chops are assumed to weigh approximately ¼ pound each, including bone.

WEIGHT MAINTENANCE MENU TABLE

Meal: Dinner Type: MD-6
Content: Rib Pork Chops
Boiled, Mashed, or Baked Potato
Half-cup Apple Sauce
Green Salad with Dressing
Bread, Beverage, and Dessert

Calorie Total	No. of Chops	Potato	Salad Dressing Tbsp.	Bread Slices	Beverage Type	Dessert Type
270	1	0	0	0	A	None
390	1	0	1	0	B	None
510	1	1	1	0	B	None
730	1	1	2	1	B	A
780	1	1	2	1	C	A
840	1	1	2	1	D	A
840	1	1	2	1	B	B
930	1	1	2	1	B	C
1030	1	1	2	1	B	D
1040	1	1	2	1	D	C
1230	1	1	2	2	D	D
490	2	0	0	0	A	None
610	2	0	1	0	B	None
730	2	1	1	1	B	None

Tabulation assumes ½ cup of apple sauce and an unlimited amount of green salad are served with each portion. Where indicated, potato is medium size and prepared with ½ pat of butter, and bread is spread with ½ pat of butter or margarine. Chops are assumed to weigh approximately ¼ pound each, including bone.

WEIGHT MAINTENANCE MENU TABLE

Meal: Dinner   Type: MD-6 (Con't)

Calorie Total	No. of Chops	Potato	Salad Dressing Tbsp.	Bread Slices	Beverage Type	Dessert Type
950	2	1	2	1	B	A
1000	2	1	2	1	C	A
1060	2	1	2	1	D	A
1060	2	1	2	1	B	B
1150	2	1	2	1	B	C
1250	2	1	2	1	B	D
1260	2	1	2	1	D	C
1450	2	1	2	2	D	D
930	4	0	0	0	A	None
1050	4	1	1	0	B	None
1170	4	1	1	0	B	None
1390	4	1	2	1	B	A
1440	4	1	2	1	C	A
1500	4	1	2	1	D	A
1500	4	1	2	1	B	B
1590	4	1	2	1	B	C
1690	4	1	2	1	B	D
1700	4	1	2	1	D	C
1890	4	1	2	2	D	D

Tabulation assumes ½ cup of apple sauce and an unlimited amount of green salad are served with each portion. Where indicated, potato is medium size and prepared with ½ pat of butter, and bread is spread with ½ pat of butter or margarine. Chops are assumed to weigh approximately ¼ pound each, including bone.

WEIGHT MAINTENANCE MENU TABLE

Meal: Dinner   Type: MD-7

Content: Roast Loin of Pork
Boiled, Mashed, or Baked Potato
Half-cup Apple Sauce
Green Salad with Dressing
Bread, Beverage, and Dessert

Calorie Total	Meat Oz.	Potato	Gravy Tbsp.	Salad Dressing Tbsp.	Bread Slices	Beverage Type	Dessert Type
390	4	0	0	0	0	A	None
510	4	0	0	1	0	B	None
630	4	1	0	1	0	B	None
890	4	1	1	2	1	B	A
980	4	1	2	2	1	C	A
1040	4	1	2	2	1	D	A
1040	4	1	2	2	1	B	B
1130	4	1	2	2	1	B	C
1230	4	1	2	2	1	B	D
1240	4	1	2	2	1	D	C
1430	4	1	2	2	2	D	D
730	8	0	0	0	0	A	None
850	8	0	0	1	0	B	None
970	8	1	0	1	0	B	None

Tabulation assumes ½ cup of apple sauce and an unlimited amount of green salad are served with each portion. Where indicated, potato is medium size and prepared with ½ pat of butter, and bread is spread with ½ pat of butter or margarine. As a guide to judging portion size, a slice of meat 4 × 4 × ¼ inch weighs approximately 4 ounces.

WEIGHT MAINTENANCE MENU TABLE

Meal: Dinner   Type: MD-7 (Con't)

Calorie Total	Meat Oz.	Potato	Gravy Tbsp.	Salad Dressing Tbsp.	Bread Slices	Beverage Type	Dessert Type
1270	8	1	2	2	1	B	A
1360	8	1	3	2	1	C	A
1420	8	1	3	2	1	D	A
1420	8	1	3	2	1	B	B
1510	8	1	3	2	1	B	C
1610	8	1	3	2	1	B	D
1620	8	1	3	2	1	D	C
1810	8	1	3	2	2	D	D
1070	12	0	0	0	0	A	None
1190	12	0	0	1	0	B	None
1310	12	1	0	1	0	B	None
1650	12	1	3	2	1	B	A
1780	12	1	5	2	1	C	A
1840	12	1	5	2	1	D	A
1840	12	1	5	2	1	B	B
1930	12	1	5	2	1	B	C
2030	12	1	5	2	1	B	D
2040	12	1	5	2	1	D	C
2230	12	1	5	2	2	D	D

Tabulation assumes ½ cup of apple sauce and an unlimited amount of green salad are served with each portion. Where indicated, potato is medium size and prepared with ½ pat of butter, and bread is spread with ½ pat of butter or margarine. As a guide to judging portion size, a slice of meat 4 × 4 × ¼ inch weighs approximately 4 ounces.

WEIGHT MAINTENANCE MENU TABLE

Meal: Dinner Type: MD-8
Content: Meat Loaf
Boiled, Mashed, or Baked Potato
Half-cup Fresh or Cooked Vegetables
Green Salad with Dressing
Bread, Beverage, and Dessert

Calorie Total	Meat Oz.	Potato	Gravy Tbsp.	Salad Dressing Tbsp.	Bread Slices	Beverage Type	Dessert Type
330	4	0	0	0	0	A	None
450	4	0	0	1	0	B	None
570	4	1	0	1	0	B	None
830	4	1	1	2	1	B	A
920	4	1	2	2	1	C	A
980	4	1	2	2	1	D	A
980	4	1	2	2	1	B	B
1070	4	1	2	2	1	B	C
1170	4	1	2	2	1	B	D
1180	4	1	2	2	1	D	C
1370	4	1	2	2	2	D	D
610	8	0	0	0	0	A	None
730	8	0	0	1	0	B	None
850	8	1	0	1	0	B	None

Tabulation assumes ½ cup of vegetables and an unlimited amount of green salad are served with each portion. Where indicated, potato is medium size and prepared with ½ pat of butter, and bread is spread with ½ pat of of butter or margarine. As a guide to judging portion size, a slice of meat loaf 3½ inches in diameter by ½ inch thick weighs approximately 4 ounces.

WEIGHT MAINTENANCE MENU TABLE

Meal: Dinner   Type: MD-8 (Con't)

Calorie Total	Meat Oz.	Potato	Gravy Tbsp.	Salad Dressing Tbsp.	Bread Slices	Beverage Type	Dessert Type
1150	8	1	2	2	1	B	A
1240	8	1	3	2	1	C	A
1300	8	1	3	2	1	D	A
1300	8	1	3	2	1	B	B
1390	8	1	3	2	1	B	C
1490	8	1	3	2	1	B	D
1500	8	1	3	2	1	D	C
1690	8	1	3	2	2	D	D
890	12	0	0	0	0	A	None
1010	12	0	0	1	0	B	None
1130	12	1	0	1	0	B	None
1470	12	1	3	2	1	B	A
1600	12	1	5	2	1	C	A
1660	12	1	5	2	1	D	A
1660	12	1	5	2	1	B	B
1750	12	1	5	2	1	B	C
1850	12	1	5	2	1	B	D
1860	12	1	5	2	1	D	C
2050	12	1	5	2	2	D	D

Tabulation assumes ½ cup of vegetables and an unlimited amount of green salad are served with each portion. Where indicated, potato is medium size and prepared with ½ pat of butter, and bread is spread with ½ pat of of butter or margarine. As a guide to judging portion size, a slice of meat loaf 3½ inches in diameter by ½ inch thick weighs approximately 4 ounces.

WEIGHT MAINTENANCE MENU TABLE

Meal: Dinner   Type: MD-9

Content: Beef and Vegetable Stew
Green Salad with Dressing
Bread, Beverage, and Dessert

Calorie Total	No. of Servings	Salad Dressing Tbsp.	Bread Slices	Beverage Type	Dessert Type
240	1	0	0	A	None
370	1	0	1	B	None
450	1	1	1	B	None
580	1	2	1	B	A
630	1	2	1	C	A
690	1	2	1	D	A
690	1	2	1	B	B
780	1	2	1	B	C
880	1	2	1	B	D
890	1	2	1	D	C
1080	1	2	2	D	D
480	2	0	0	A	None
610	2	0	1	B	None
690	2	1	1	B	None
820	2	2	1	B	A

A serving of stew consists of one cup of meat (approximately 2 ounces), vegetables, potatoes, and gravy. Where bread is indicated, it is spread with ½ pat of butter or margarine. An unlimited amount of green salad may be eaten without significantly increasing the calorie totals.

WEIGHT MAINTENANCE MENU TABLE

Meal: Dinner   Type: MD-9 (Con't)

Calorie Total	No. of Servings	Salad Dressing Tbsp.	Bread Slices	Beverage Type	Dessert Type
870	2	2	1	C	A
930	2	2	1	D	A
930	2	2	1	B	B
1020	2	2	1	B	C
1120	2	2	1	B	D
1130	2	2	1	D	C
1320	2	2	2	D	D
720	3	0	0	A	None
850	3	0	1	B	None
930	3	1	1	B	None
1060	3	2	1	B	A
1110	3	2	1	C	A
1170	3	2	1	D	A
1170	3	2	1	B	B
1260	3	2	1	B	C
1360	3	2	1	B	D
1370	3	2	1	D	C
1560	3	2	2	D	D

A serving of stew consists of one cup of meat (approximately 2 ounces), vegetables, potatoes, and gravy. Where bread is indicated, it is spread with ½ pat of butter or margarine. An unlimited amount of green salad may be eaten without significantly increasing the calorie totals.

WEIGHT MAINTENANCE MENU TABLE

Meal: Dinner   Type: MD-10

Content: Roast Chicken or Turkey
Boiled, Mashed, or Baked Potato
Half-cup Fresh or Cooked Vegetables
Green Salad with Dressing
Bread, Beverage, and Dessert

Calorie Total	Meat Oz.	Potato	Gravy Tbsp.	Salad Dressing Tbsp.	Bread Slices	Beverage Type	Dessert Type
290	4	0	0	0	0	A	None
410	4	0	0	1	0	B	None
530	4	1	0	1	0	B	None
790	4	1	1	2	1	B	A
880	4	1	2	2	1	C	A
940	4	1	2	2	1	D	A
940	4	1	2	2	1	B	B
1030	4	1	2	2	1	B	C
1130	4	1	2	2	1	B	D
1140	4	1	2	2	1	D	C
1330	4	1	2	2	2	D	D
530	8	0	0	0	0	A	None
650	8	0	0	1	0	B	None
770	8	1	0	1	0	B	None

Tabulation assumes ½ cup of vegetables and an unlimited amount of green salad are served with each portion. Where indicated, potato is prepared with ½ pat of butter, and bread is spread with ½ pat of butter or margarine. As a guide to judging portion size, the average drumstick contains 2 ounces of meat, while ½ a breast has approximately 3 ounces.

WEIGHT MAINTENANCE MENU TABLE

Meal: Dinner   Type: MD-10 (Con't)

Calorie Total	Meat Oz.	Potato	Gravy Tbsp.	Salad Dressing Tbsp.	Bread Slices	Beverage Type	Dessert Type
1070	8	1	2	2	1	B	A
1160	8	1	3	2	1	C	A
1220	8	1	3	2	1	D	A
1220	8	1	3	2	1	B	B
1310	8	1	3	2	1	B	C
1410	8	1	3	2	1	B	D
1420	8	1	3	2	1	D	C
1610	8	1	3	2	2	D	D
770	12	0	0	0	0	A	None
890	12	0	0	1	0	B	None
1010	12	1	0	1	0	B	None
1350	12	1	3	2	1	B	A
1480	12	1	5	2	1	C	A
1540	12	1	5	2	1	D	A
1540	12	1	5	2	1	B	B
1630	12	1	5	2	1	B	C
1730	12	1	5	2	1	B	D
1740	12	1	5	2	1	D	C
1930	12	1	5	2	2	D	D

Tabulation assumes ½ cup of vegetables and an unlimited amount of green salad are served with each portion. Where indicated, potato is prepared with ½ pat of butter, and bread is spread with ½ pat of butter or margarine. As a guide to judging portion size, the average drumstick contains 2 ounces of meat, while ½ a breast has approximately 3 ounces.

WEIGHT MAINTENANCE MENU TABLE

Meal: Dinner   Type: MD-11

Content: Breaded and Fried Chicken
Boiled, Mashed, or Baked Potato
Half-cup Fresh or Cooked Vegetables
Green Salad with Dressing
Bread, Beverage, and Dessert

Calorie Total	Meat Oz.	Potato	Salad Dressing Tbsp.	Bread Slices	Beverage Type	Dessert Type
350	4	0	0	0	A	None
470	4	0	1	0	B	None
590	4	1	1	0	B	None
810	4	1	2	1	B	A
860	4	1	2	1	C	A
920	4	1	2	1	D	A
920	4	1	2	1	B	B
1010	4	1	2	1	B	C
1110	4	1	2	1	B	D
1120	4	1	2	1	D	C
1310	4	1	2	2	D	D
650	8	0	0	0	A	None
770	8	0	1	0	B	None
890	8	1	1	0	B	None

Tabulation assumes ½ cup of vegetables and an unlimited amount of green salad are served with each portion. Where indicated, potato is prepared with ½ pat of butter, and bread is spread with ½ pat of butter or margarine. As a guide to judging portion size, the average drumstick contains 2 ounces of meat, while ½ a breast has approximately 3 ounces.

WEIGHT MAINTENANCE MENU TABLE

Meal: Dinner   Type: MD-11 (Con't)

Calorie Total	Meat Oz.	Potato	Salad Dressing Tbsp.	Bread Slices	Beverage Type	Dessert Type
1110	8	1	2	1	B	A
1160	8	1	2	1	C	A
1220	8	1	2	1	D	A
1220	8	1	2	1	B	B
1310	8	1	2	1	B	C
1410	8	1	2	1	B	D
1420	8	1	2	1	D	C
1610	8	1	2	2	D	D
950	12	0	0	0	A	None
1070	12	0	1	0	B	None
1190	12	1	1	0	B	None
1410	12	1	2	1	B	A
1460	12	1	2	1	C	A
1520	12	1	2	1	D	A
1520	12	1	2	1	B	B
1610	12	1	2	1	B	C
1710	12	1	2	1	B	D
1720	12	1	2	1	D	C
1910	12	1	2	2	D	D

Tabulation assumes ½ cup of vegetables and an unlimited amount of green salad are served with each portion. Where indicated, potato is prepared with ½ pat of butter, and bread is spread with ½ pat of butter or margarine. As a guide to judging portion size, the average drumstick contains 2 ounces of meat, while ½ a breast has approximately 3 ounces.

WEIGHT MAINTENANCE MENU TABLE

Meal: Dinner Type: MD-12

Content: Braised Chicken with Vegetables Casserole
Boiled Rice
Green Salad with Dressing
Bread, Beverage, and Dessert

Calorie Total	No. of Servings	Rice Cups	Salad Dressing Tbsp.	Bread Slices	Beverage Type	Dessert Type
200	1	0	0	0	A	None
320	1	0	1	0	B	None
430	1	1/2	1	0	B	None
650	1	1/2	2	1	B	A
700	1	1/2	2	1	C	A
760	1	1/2	2	1	D	A
760	1	1/2	2	1	B	B
850	1	1/2	2	1	B	C
950	1	1/2	2	1	B	D
960	1	1/2	2	1	D	C
1150	1	1/2	2	2	D	D
400	2	0	0	0	A	None
520	2	0	1	0	B	None
740	2	1	1	0	B	None

A casserole serving consists of one cup of chicken (approximately 2 ounces), vegetables, and gravy. Where bread is indicated, it is spread with ½ pat of butter or margarine. An unlimited amount of green salad may be eaten without significantly increasing the calorie totals. As a guide to judging portion size, the average drumstick contains 2 ounces of meat, while ½ a breast has approximately 3 ounces.

WEIGHT MAINTENANCE MENU TABLE

Meal: Dinner   Type: MD-12 (Con't)

Calorie Total	No. of Servings	Rice Cups	Salad Dressing Tbsp.	Bread Slices	Beverage Type	Dessert Type
960	2	1	2	1	B	A
1010	2	1	2	1	C	A
1070	2	1	2	1	D	A
1070	2	1	2	1	B	B
1160	2	1	2	1	B	C
1260	2	1	2	1	B	D
1270	2	1	2	1	D	C
1460	2	1	2	2	D	D
600	3	0	0	0	A	None
720	3	0	1	0	B	None
1050	3	1½	1	0	B	None
1270	3	1½	2	1	B	A
1320	3	1½	2	1	C	A
1380	3	1½	2	1	D	A
1380	3	1½	2	1	B	B
1470	3	1½	2	1	B	C
1570	3	1½	2	1	B	D
1580	3	1½	2	1	D	C
1770	3	1½	2	2	D	D

A casserole serving consists of one cup of chicken (approximately 2 ounces), vegetables, and gravy. Where bread is indicated, it is spread with ½ pat of butter or margarine. An unlimited amount of green salad may be eaten without significantly increasing the calorie totals. As a guide to judging portion size, the average drumstick contains 2 ounces of meat, while ½ a breast has approximately 3 ounces.

WEIGHT MAINTENANCE MENU TABLE

Meal: Dinner   Type: MD-13

Content: Roast Duck, Orange Sauce
Wild Rice
Half-cup Fresh or Cooked Vegetables
Green Salad with Dressing
Bread, Beverage, and Dessert

Calorie Total	Meat Oz.	Rice Cups	Salad Dressing Tbsp.	Bread Slices	Beverage Type	Dessert Type
430	4	0	0	0	A	None
550	4	0	1	0	B	None
660	4	1/2	1	0	B	None
880	4	1/2	2	1	B	A
930	4	1/2	2	1	C	A
990	4	1/2	2	1	D	A
990	4	1/2	2	1	B	B
1080	4	1/2	2	1	B	C
1180	4	1/2	2	1	B	D
1190	4	1/2	2	1	D	C
1380	4	1/2	2	2	D	D
810	8	0	0	0	A	None
930	8	0	1	0	B	None
1150	8	1	1	0	B	None

Tabulation assumes ½ cup of vegetables and an unlimited amount of green salad are served with each portion. Where indicated, potato is prepared with ½ pat of butter, and bread is spread with ½ pat of butter or margarine. As a guide to judging portion size, the average drumstick contains 2 ounces of meat, while ½ a breast has approximately 3 ounces.

WEIGHT MAINTENANCE MENU TABLE
Meal: Dinner   Type: MD-13 (Con't)

Calorie Total	Meat Oz.	Rice Cups	Salad Dressing Tbsp.	Bread Slices	Beverage Type	Dessert Type
1370	8	1	2	1	B	A
1420	8	1	2	1	C	A
1480	8	1	2	1	D	A
1480	8	1	2	1	B	B
1570	8	1	2	1	B	C
1670	8	1	2	1	B	D
1680	8	1	2	1	D	C
1870	8	1	2	2	D	D
1190	12	0	0	0	A	None
1310	12	0	1	0	B	None
1530	12	1	1	0	B	None
1750	12	1	2	1	B	A
1800	12	1	2	1	C	A
1860	12	1	2	1	D	A
1860	12	1	2	1	B	B
1950	12	1	2	1	B	C
2050	12	1	2	1	B	D
2060	12	1	2	1	D	C
2250	12	1	2	2	D	D

Tabulation assumes ½ cup of vegetables and an unlimited amount of green salad are served with each portion. Where indicated, potato is prepared with ½ pat of butter, and bread is spread with ½ pat of butter or margarine. As a guide to judging portion size, the average drumstick contains 2 ounces of meat, while ½ a breast has approximately 3 ounces.

WEIGHT MAINTENANCE MENU TABLE

Meal: Dinner   Type: MD-14

Content: Fish, Baked or Broiled
         Boiled, Mashed, or Baked
           Potato
         Half-cup Fresh or Cooked
           Vegetables
         Green Salad with Dressing
         Bread, Beverage, and Dessert

Calorie Total	Fish Oz.	Potato	Salad Dressing Tbsp.	Bread Slices	Beverage Type	Dessert Type
250	4	0	0	0	A	None
370	4	0	1	0	B	None
490	4	1	1	0	B	None
710	4	1	2	1	B	A
760	4	1	2	1	C	A
820	4	1	2	1	D	A
820	4	1	2	1	B	B
910	4	1	2	1	B	C
1010	4	1	2	1	B	D
1020	4	1	2	1	D	C
1210	4	1	2	2	D	D
450	8	0	0	0	A	None
570	8	0	1	0	B	None
690	8	1	1	0	B	None

Tabulation assumes ½ cup of vegetables and an unlimited amount of green salad are served with each portion. Where indicated, potato is prepared with ½ pat of butter, and bread is spread with ½ pat of butter or margarine. As a guide to judging portion size, a section of fish 4 × 4 × ¼ inch weighs approximately 4 ounces.

WEIGHT MAINTENANCE MENU TABLE

Meal: Dinner   Type: MD-14 (Con't)

Calorie Total	Fish Oz.	Potato	Salad Dressing Tbsp.	Bread Slices	Beverage Type	Dessert Type
910	8	1	2	1	B	A
960	8	1	2	1	C	A
1020	8	1	2	1	D	A
1020	8	1	2	1	B	B
1110	8	1	2	1	B	C
1210	8	1	2	1	B	D
1220	8	1	2	1	D	C
1410	8	1	2	2	D	D
850	12	0	0	0	A	None
970	12	0	1	0	B	None
1090	12	1	1	0	B	None
1310	12	1	2	1	B	A
1360	12	1	2	1	C	A
1420	12	1	2	1	D	A
1420	12	1	2	1	B	B
1510	12	1	2	1	B	C
1610	12	1	2	1	B	D
1620	12	1	2	1	D	C
1810	12	1	2	2	D	D

Tabulation assumes ½ cup of vegetables and an unlimited amount of green salad are served with each portion. Where indicated, potato is prepared with ½ pat of butter, and bread is spread with ½ pat of butter or margarine. As a guide to judging portion size, a section of fish 4 × 4 × ¼ inch weighs approximately 4 ounces.

WEIGHT MAINTENANCE MENU TABLE

Meal: Dinner Type: MD-15
Content: Breaded and Fried Fish
Boiled, Mashed, or Baked Potato
Half-cup Fresh or Cooked Vegetables
Green Salad with Dressing
Bread, Beverage, and Dessert

Calorie Total	Fish Oz.	Potato	Salad Dressing Tbsp.	Bread Slices	Beverage Type	Dessert Type
310	4	0	0	0	A	None
430	4	0	1	0	B	None
550	4	1	1	0	B	None
770	4	1	2	1	B	A
820	4	1	2	1	C	A
880	4	1	2	1	D	A
880	4	1	2	1	B	B
970	4	1	2	1	B	C
1070	4	1	2	1	B	D
1080	4	1	2	1	D	C
1270	4	1	2	2	D	D
570	8	0	0	0	A	None
690	8	0	1	0	B	None
810	8	1	1	0	B	None

Tabulation assumes ½ cup of vegetables and an unlimited amount of green salad are served with each portion. Where indicated, potato is prepared with ½ pat of butter, and bread is spread with ½ pat of butter or margarine. As a guide to judging portion size, a section of fish 4 × 4 × ¼ inch weighs approximately 4 ounces.

WEIGHT MAINTENANCE MENU TABLE

Meal: Dinner   Type: MD-15 (Con't)

Calorie Total	Fish Oz.	Potato	Salad Dressing Tbsp.	Bread Slices	Beverage Type	Dessert Type
1030	8	1	2	1	B	A
1080	8	1	2	1	C	A
1140	8	1	2	1	D	A
1140	8	1	2	1	B	B
1230	8	1	2	1	B	C
1330	8	1	2	1	B	D
1340	8	1	2	1	D	C
1530	8	1	2	2	D	D
830	12	0	0	0	A	None
950	12	0	1	0	B	None
1070	12	1	1	0	B	None
1290	12	1	2	1	B	A
1340	12	1	2	1	C	A
1400	12	1	2	1	D	A
1400	12	1	2	1	B	B
1490	12	1	2	1	B	C
1590	12	1	2	1	B	D
1600	12	1	2	1	D	C
1790	12	1	2	2	D	D

Tabulation assumes ½ cup of vegetables and an unlimited amount of green salad are served with each portion. Where indicated, potato is prepared with ½ pat of butter, and bread is spread with ½ pat of butter or margarine. As a guide to judging portion size, a section of fish 4 × 4 × ¼ inch weighs approximately 4 ounces.

WEIGHT MAINTENANCE MENU TABLE

Meal: Dinner Type: MD-16
Content: Seafood Gumbo
Boiled Rice
Green Salad with Dressing
Bread, Beverage, and Dessert

Calorie Total	No. of Servings	Rice Cups	Salad Dressing Tbsp.	Bread Slices	Beverage Type	Dessert Type
160	1	0	0	0	A	None
280	1	0	1	0	B	None
390	1	1/2	1	0	B	None
610	1	1/2	2	1	B	A
660	1	1/2	2	1	C	A
720	1	1/2	2	1	D	A
720	1	1/2	2	1	B	B
810	1	1/2	2	1	B	C
910	1	1/2	2	1	B	D
920	1	1/2	2	1	D	C
1110	1	1/2	2	2	D	D
320	2	0	0	0	A	None
440	2	0	1	0	B	None
660	2	1	1	0	B	None
880	2	1	2	1	B	A

A serving of seafood gumbo consists of one cup of fish (approximately 2 ounces of any kind), vegetables, and sauce. Where bread is indicated, it is spread with ½ pat of butter or margarine. An unlimited amount of green salad may be eaten without significantly increasing the calorie totals.

WEIGHT MAINTENANCE MENU TABLE

Meal: Dinner   Type: MD-16 (Con't)

Calorie Total	No. of Servings	Rice Cups	Salad Dressing Tbsp.	Bread Slices	Beverage Type	Dessert Type
930	2	1	2	1	C	A
990	2	1	2	1	D	A
990	2	1	2	1	B	B
1080	2	1	2	1	B	C
1180	2	1	2	1	B	D
1190	2	1	2	1	D	C
1380	2	1	2	2	D	D
480	3	0	0	0	A	None
600	3	0	1	0	B	None
930	3	1½	1	0	B	None
1150	3	1½	2	1	B	A
1200	3	1½	2	1	C	A
1260	3	1½	2	1	D	A
1260	3	1½	2	1	B	B
1350	3	1½	2	1	B	C
1450	3	1½	2	1	B	D
1460	3	1½	2	1	D	C
1650	3	1½	2	2	D	D

A serving of seafood gumbo consists of one cup of fish (approximately 2 ounces of any kind), vegetables, and sauce. Where bread is indicated, it is spread with ½ pat of butter or margarine. An unlimited amount of green salad may be eaten without significantly increasing the calorie totals.

WEIGHT MAINTENANCE MENU TABLE

Meal: Dinner   Type: MD-17

Content: Lobster, Boiled or Steamed
           Clam Chowder
           Boiled or Baked Potato
           Half-cup Fresh or Cooked
              Vegetables
           Green Salad with Dressing
           Bread, Beverage, and Dessert

Calorie Total	No. of Lobsters	Soup Cups	Potato	Salad Dressing Tbsp.	Bread Slices	Beverage Type	Dessert Type
270	1	0	0	0	0	A	None
340	1	0	0	1	0	B	None
590	1	0	1	2	0	B	A
780	1	0	1	2	1	C	A
840	1	0	1	2	1	D	A
1030	1	0	1	2	1	B	D
1040	1	0	1	2	1	D	C
1140	1	0	1	2	1	D	D
470	1	1	0	0	0	A	None
540	1	1	0	1	0	B	None
790	1	1	1	2	0	B	A
980	1	1	1	2	1	C	A
1040	1	1	1	2	1	D	A

Tabulation assumes ½ cup of vegetables and an unlimited amount of green salad are served with each portion. Where indicated, potato is prepared with ½ pat of butter, and bread is spread with ½ pat of butter or margarine. Clam chowder is assumed to be New England (white) style, and lobster is assumed to weigh 1¼ lbs.

WEIGHT MAINTENANCE MENU TABLE

Meal: Dinner   Type: MD-17 (Con't)

Calorie Total	No. of Lobsters	Soup Cups	Potato	Salad Dressing Tbsp.	Bread Slices	Beverage Type	Dessert Type
1230	1	1	1	2	1	B	D
1240	1	1	1	2	1	D	C
1340	1	1	1	2	1	D	D
490	2	0	0	0	0	A	None
560	2	0	0	1	0	B	None
810	2	0	1	2	0	B	A
1000	2	0	1	2	1	C	A
1060	2	0	1	2	1	D	A
1250	2	0	1	2	1	B	D
1260	2	0	1	2	1	D	C
1360	2	0	1	2	1	D	D
690	2	1	0	0	0	A	None
760	2	1	0	1	0	B	None
1010	2	1	1	2	0	B	A
1200	2	1	1	2	1	C	A
1260	2	1	1	2	1	D	A
1450	2	1	1	2	1	B	D
1460	2	1	1	2	1	D	C
1560	2	1	1	2	1	D	D

Tabulation assumes ½ cup of vegetables and an unlimited amount of green salad are served with each portion. Where indicated, potato is prepared with ½ pat of butter, and bread is spread with ½ pat of butter or margarine. Clam chowder is assumed to be New England (white) style, and lobster is assumed to weigh 1¼ lbs.

WEIGHT MAINTENANCE MENU TABLE

Meal: Dinner   Type: MD-18

Content: Broiled Shrimp
          Boiled, Mashed, or Baked
             Potato
          Half-cup Fresh or Cooked
             Vegetables
          Green Salad with Dressing
          Bread, Beverage, and Dessert

Calorie Total	Shrimp Oz.	Potato	Salad Dressing Tbsp.	Bread Slices	Beverage Type	Dessert Type
230	4	0	0	0	A	None
350	4	0	1	0	B	None
470	4	1	1	0	B	None
690	4	1	2	1	B	A
740	4	1	2	1	C	A
800	4	1	2	1	D	A
800	4	1	2	1	B	B
890	4	1	2	1	B	C
990	4	1	2	1	B	D
1000	4	1	2	1	D	C
1190	4	1	2	2	D	D
410	8	0	0	0	A	None
530	8	0	1	0	B	None
650	8	1	1	0	B	None

Tabulation assumes ½ cup of vegetables and an unlimited amount of green salad are served with each portion. Where indicated, potato is prepared with ½ pat of butter, and bread is spread with ½ pat of butter or margarine. As a guide to judging portion size, 6 medium size shrimp weigh approximately 4 ounces.

WEIGHT MAINTENANCE MENU TABLE

Meal: Dinner   Type: MD-18 (Con't)

Calorie Total	Shrimp Oz.	Potato	Salad Dressing Tbsp.	Bread Slices	Beverage Type	Dessert Type
870	8	1	2	1	B	A
920	8	1	2	1	C	A
980	8	1	2	1	D	A
980	8	1	2	1	B	B
1070	8	1	2	1	B	C
1170	8	1	2	1	B	D
1180	8	1	2	1	D	C
1370	8	1	2	2	D	D
590	12	0	0	0	A	None
710	12	0	1	0	B	None
830	12	1	1	0	B	None
1050	12	1	2	1	B	A
1100	12	1	2	1	C	A
1160	12	1	2	1	D	A
1160	12	1	2	1	B	B
1250	12	1	2	1	B	C
1350	12	1	2	1	B	D
1360	12	1	2	1	D	C
1550	12	1	2	2	D	D

Tabulation assumes ½ cup of vegetables and an unlimited amount of green salad are served with each portion. Where indicated, potato is prepared with ½ pat of butter, and bread is spread with ½ pat of butter or margarine. As a guide to judging portion size, 6 medium size shrimp weigh approximately 4 ounces.

WEIGHT MAINTENANCE MENU TABLE

Meal: Dinner Type: MD-19

Content: Macaroni and Cheese Casserole
Half-cup Fresh or Cooked Vegetables
Green Salad with Dressing
Bread, Beverage, and Dessert

Calorie Total	Casserole Cups	Salad Dressing Tbsp.	Bread Slices	Beverage Type	Dessert Type
480	1	0	0	A	None
600	1	1	0	B	None
650	1	1	0	C	None
770	1	2	1	B	A
820	1	2	1	C	A
880	1	2	1	D	A
880	1	2	1	B	B
970	1	2	1	B	C
1070	1	2	1	B	D
1080	1	2	1	D	C
1270	1	2	2	D	D
910	2	0	0	A	None
1030	2	1	0	B	None
1080	2	1	0	C	None

Tabulation assumes ½ cup of vegetables and an unlimited amount of green salad are served with each portion. Where bread is indicated, it is spread with ½ pat of butter or margarine.

WEIGHT MAINTENANCE MENU TABLE

Meal: Dinner   Type: MD-19 (Con't)

Calorie Total	Casserole Cups	Salad Dressing Tbsp.	Bread Slices	Beverage Type	Dessert Type
1200	2	2	1	B	A
1250	2	2	1	C	A
1310	2	2	1	D	A
1310	2	2	1	B	B
1400	2	2	1	B	C
1500	2	2	1	B	D
1510	2	2	1	D	C
1700	2	2	2	D	D
1340	3	0	0	A	None
1460	3	1	0	B	None
1510	3	1	0	C	None
1630	3	2	1	B	A
1680	3	2	1	C	A
1740	3	2	1	D	A
1740	3	2	1	B	B
1830	3	2	1	B	C
1930	3	2	1	B	D
1940	3	2	1	D	C
2130	3	2	2	D	D

Tabulation assumes ½ cup of vegetables and an unlimited amount of green salad are served with each portion. Where bread is indicated, it is spread with ½ pat of butter or margarine.

WEIGHT MAINTENANCE MENU TABLE

Meal: Dinner   Type: MD-20

Content: Spaghetti, Tomato Sauce
Meat Balls
Green Salad with Dressing
Bread, Beverage, and Dessert

Calorie Total	Spaghetti Servings	Meat Balls	Salad Dressing Tbsp.	Bread Slices	Beverage Type	Dessert Type
220	1	0	0	0	A	None
340	1	0	1	0	B	None
560	1	0	2	1	B	A
610	1	0	2	1	C	A
670	1	0	2	1	D	A
860	1	0	2	1	B	D
870	1	0	2	1	D	C
1060	1	0	2	2	D	D
480	1	2	0	0	A	None
600	1	2	1	0	B	None
820	1	2	2	1	B	A
870	1	2	2	1	C	A
930	1	2	2	1	D	A
1120	1	2	2	1	B	D

Tabulation assumes an unlimited amount of green salad is served with each portion. A serving of spaghetti contains one cup of cooked pasta, with 6 tbsp. of tomato sauce and a liberal sprinkling of cheese. Meat balls are assumed to weigh approximately 2 ounces each.

WEIGHT MAINTENANCE MENU TABLE

Meal: Dinner   Type: MD-20 (Con't)

Calorie Total	Spaghetti Servings	Meat Balls	Salad Dressing Tbsp.	Bread Slices	Beverage Type	Dessert Type
1130	1	2	2	1	D	C
1320	1	2	2	2	D	D
440	2	0	0	0	A	None
560	2	0	1	0	B	None
780	2	0	2	1	B	A
830	2	0	2	1	C	A
890	2	0	2	1	D	A
1080	2	0	2	1	B	D
1090	2	0	2	1	D	C
1280	2	0	2	2	D	D
960	2	4	0	0	A	None
1080	2	4	1	0	B	None
1300	2	4	2	1	B	A
1440	2	4	2	2	C	A
1500	2	4	2	2	D	A
1690	2	4	2	2	B	D
1700	2	4	2	2	D	C
1800	2	4	2	2	D	D

Tabulation assumes an unlimited amount of green salad is served with each portion. A serving of spaghetti contains one cup of cooked pasta, with 6 tbsp. of tomato sauce and a liberal sprinkling of cheese. Meat balls are assumed to weigh approximately 2 ounces each.

10. Planning a Weight Maintenance Program

Seventy days have passed since our imaginary friend started her diet. She has lost fifteen pounds, and has already determined, from the Weight Maintenance Calorie Tables that, in order to maintain her weight at 125 pounds, she must restrict her food intake to approximately 2250 calories per day. She now proceeds in much the same way as when she planned her weight loss diet.

Weekly Routine: Her total weekly caloric allowance is 15,750 calories (7 × 2250). She anticipates continued overeating problems on weekends, and decides to allow an extra 1000 calories for the weekend. As a result, her maintenance values become 2050 calories per day on weekdays, and 2750 calories per day on weekends.

Daily Routine: In this example, we will only consider the 2050 calorie weekday meals. Let us assume she decides to split the day's calories as follows:

Breakfast	400
Mid-morning snack	150
Lunch	400
Dinner	900
Evening snack	200
	2050 calories

She is now ready to use the Weight Maintenance Menu Tables to establish the eating plan she is going to observe for the foreseeable future. Her meals for a weekday could be the following:

MB-1: One cup of fresh strawberries, a scrambled egg with two strips of bacon, one slice of buttered toast, and a cup of coffee with milk and sugar. (390 calories)

DL-4:* 4 ounces of tuna (oil-packed), ½ cup of green beans, one slice of enriched bread, and 4 ounces of skim milk (no dessert). (370 calories)

MD-10: 4 ounces of roast chicken, baked potato with butter, 2 tbsp. gravy, green salad with 2 tbsp. dressing, one slice of buttered bread, a small glass of wine, and one cookie. (890 calories)

The mid-morning snack could be a cup of coffee and a plain donut (175 calories), with an evening snack of a cup of flavored yogurt (250 calories). The total for the day is 2065 calories.

At this point, you have all of the information you need to plan your own maintenance eating plan.

Monitoring Calories

All the hints given regarding calorie control during a reducing diet can be used on your maintenance program; that is, allocate a definite calorie count for each meal, monitor only the calories eaten at each meal, and use the Set Meal concept for one or two of your daily meals.

However, it is a fact of life that no matter how determined one is to abide by an eating plan, events have a way of forcing deviation. The way to handle these occurrences is by compensating. The art of compensating is

---

* A diet lunch was chosen (and you certainly may select a diet meal, even on maintenance) because a 400 calorie allowance for lunch is quite low.

achieved by estimating how far you have strayed from your plan and making amends at the next opportunity (usually the next meal)—by eating less.

For example, let us say you are obliged to attend a business luncheon. Furthermore, assume that the meal has been pre-ordered and you have no choice but to eat what is served. Do so, but at some point toward the end of the meal mentally estimate the number of calories you have eaten. Suppose the total was approximately 900 calories. If your normal set lunch is 500 calories, you know you have overeaten by 400 calories. Right then, you might decide to have water as your dinner beverage and to eliminate your evening snack. By doing this, you would have compensated, before the end of the day, for the extra 400 calories you ate at lunch.

Finally, I recommend that on a maintenance regimen you "weigh in" once a week. You should do this at the same time of the day, on the same scale, and preferably unclothed. If a weight gain of more than three pounds is noticed, immediately revert to a weight loss diet until the added weight is lost.

Weight Maintenance Summarized

The following is the step-by-step procedure you should follow to develop a customized *weight maintenance plan.*

Step 1. Find your Activity Level from the table on page 14.

Step 2. From the Weight Maintenance Calorie Table Index on page 129, locate the table that applies to you.

Step 3. Use your Weight Maintenance Calorie Table to determine how many calories you may eat per day.

Step 4. Allocate your calorie total among the days of the week.
Step 5. Allocate your calorie allowance among the meals of the day.
Step 6. Determine which of the meals of the day will be Set Meals.
Step 7. Consult the Weight Maintenance Menu Tables (Index on page 147) and plan your Set Meals.

Also use the Weight Maintenance Menu Tables to plan a meal pattern for an entire day. This will give you a good idea of the type of portion sizes you are allowed.

11. They Did It—You Can Too!

There is no one right way to solve the weight control problems that afflict millions of people. It is my opinion, however, that the data presented in this book, if applied with judgment, can provide the basis for designing a personalized weight control program for virtually any situation. My purpose here is to illustrate the application of this book to everyday weight control problems* as well as the variations in approach that are possible.

65, Retired, and Overweight

The first example concerns a retired schoolteacher. In her younger days she was quite active. She is a friend of my mother, and I remember that she was a fine tennis player and an enthusiastic hiker. As she told it, "I used to be able to eat anything, and I never gained a pound!"

There were two reasons for her weight gain. The first was her lack of activity. (About five years ago, she injured her hip in an accident, and now walks with a cane.) The second reason was her slowly decreasing

---

* The weight control experiences that follow are based on real people and situations. However, I have purposely combined some events and used fictitious names, ages, occupations, and weights in order to avoid identification. Any similarity to persons known or unknown to me is purely coincidental.

basal metabolic rate, which happens to all of us with advancing age (page 40, axiom 5).

She had not compensated for these factors; that is, she had not changed her eating habits and, as a consequence, she was overweight and unhappy about it.

During the Christmas holidays she confided in me that she had gone to a doctor she had heard about through a friend. "He gave me an examination," she said, "and a diet to follow, and then prescriptions for pills."

I knew the pill routine—a diuretic for a quick loss of water (which the patient interprets as a "real" weight loss), an appetite suppressant, and a thyroid medication to increase the metabolic rate. For some people, the side effects of this type of treatment can be pretty bad.

"I became a nervous wreck," she continued. "First, I couldn't sleep. Then he gave me more pills. I finally stopped taking the pills. I quickly regained the few pounds I had lost [the water weight], and I was back to where I started."

I asked if the doctor had found any medical problems during his examination.

"No. He said I was in good health but that I should lose thirty pounds."

She knew I was writing a book on the subject and asked if I could help. When I returned home and had access to my tables, I wrote her a long letter suggesting what she should do.

I knew her age, but she wouldn't tell me her exact weight! I guessed that she was close to 160 pounds, and about 5′ 5″ tall. In order to lose 30 pounds at the recommended rate of two pounds per week, she had to allow 15 weeks or 105 days for her diet. I estimated her Activity Level to be between 0 and 1. Therefore, the Weight Loss Calorie Tables that apply to her are on pages 88 and 89. Interpolating between the values on these pages, I found that on a 1200 calorie diet it would take her approximately 135 days to lose 30 pounds.

My mother gave me periodic "progress reports." She said her friend was delighted with the diet and was happily losing weight. After some five months, however, I got a phone call.

"I lost the 30 pounds, but I have already gained five pounds back!"

My fault! I had neglected to give her maintenance instructions. I recommended she revert to the 1200 calorie diet, and the next time I saw her, we talked maintenance.

The Overweight Weightlifter

Greg wanted to compete in the 198 pound class. He was 25 years old, 6′ 1″, and 220 pounds. The meet was one month away.

I had gone to school with his older brother, and the three of us usually jogged together. It was while jogging that Greg related his problem. ". . . I know I can win the 198 pound class," he said, "but I don't want to train for a month and then miss the weight."

We met that night to map our strategy. Greg is a surveyor, and because he is so active, his normal Activity Level is at least 2. When he trains for an event, he works out five days a week (2½ hours each day), and I would conservatively estimate his Activity Level at 3. We figured that if he could lose 20 pounds, he would be close enough to his goal to "sweat-off" any remaining weight just before weigh-in time. The Weight Loss Calorie Table on page 70 showed that if Greg went on a 1500 calorie diet, he would lose 20 pounds in 29 days.

The 1500 calorie diet he followed was almost identical to that shown in Appendix A, except that Greg substituted 4 ounces of skim milk wherever coffee with milk and sugar was specified.

The night before the weigh-in, his weight was 201 pounds. By restricting his fluid intake and spending some time in the steam room immediately prior to the weigh-in, he came in at 196 pounds. Of course, after a good meal and two glasses of milk, he actually competed at 201 pounds—a procedure not uncommon in sports competition.

After the competition, Greg decided he felt better at 200 pounds than he did at his higher weight level. Here is how he went about stabilizing his weight at 200 pounds. Referring to the Weight Maintenance Calorie Table on page 136, we found that when he weighed 220 pounds he must have been consuming 3680 calories per day, and to remain at 200 pounds, with an Activity Level of 2, he would have to cut back his caloric intake to 3460.

He saw the trend of my reasoning and said, "Oh no, I don't want to keep counting calories."

"You don't have to," I replied. "What you should do is examine what you usually ate at 220 pounds, and deduct 220 (3680 − 3460) calories per day. You don't have to count calories!"

I asked him to write down exactly what he had eaten in a typical day before he started on his reducing diet.

"Good, now let's trim 220 calories."

The foods trimmed must be items you eat every day. In this way, when you eliminate them, you eliminate known calories. In Greg's case, this amounted to eliminating a slice of buttered toast from breakfast (90 calories) and a can of beer (150 calories) which he drank after his workouts.

This last point illustrates another method you can use to maintain your weight after a reducing diet. That is, use the Weight Maintenance Calorie Tables to calculate the difference between the maintenance calories required to sustain your weight at the start and the end of a reducing diet, and then eliminate that number of calories from your pre-reducing eating pattern.

Since we are discussing athletes, it is interesting to note why so many athletes gain weight in the off-season or after they retire from active competition. Assume that Greg was a professional athlete. (He is big enough to have been a football player.) If his playing weight was 220 pounds and his Activity Level was 3, his maintenance calorie needs would be 4220 calories per day (page 136). Then he stops competing—he retires. His activity level drops to 2 (he had better play a lot of golf, because even this is quite high). If he continues to eat as he did while an active professional (4220 calories), he will naturally gain weight.

How much? Greg's weight will slowly rise (about one pound a week) until it reaches approximately 270 pounds. He will stop gaining at 270 pounds because, according to the Weight Maintenance Calorie Table, at that weight his calorie needs will be approximately 4200 calories, which balances his food calorie intake.

She Works in a Bakery!

I dread the thought of what I might weigh if I worked in a bakery! Well, I went to grammar school with a girl who, with her husband, now operates a bakery in my hometown.

They Did It—You Can Too! 221

I was visiting my mother, and went to the bakery on a Sunday morning to buy some breakfast rolls.

"I hear you're writing a diet book," said her husband, Al.

My mother really gets around, I thought. "Yes," I answered.

"If you can get Doris to reduce, I'll give your mother free rolls for a year!"

"Something's wrong with my glands!" Doris declared. "I hardly eat anything and I still gain weight."

"If you have a minute," I said, "tell me what you eat in a normal day."

"For breakfast, I have toast and coffee, and for lunch. . . ."

I asked questions about quantity, food preparation, etc. Using my mental "ballpark" calorie table, I estimated her calorie total at 1900. Too little to account for her weight.

"What else do you eat? What about this delicious cake?"

"I have a few pieces during the day—just to see if they're fresh. It doesn't amount to much."

"How many?"

"Well, I usually have a cheese danish with my coffee at 9 A.M., then right after. . . ."

Amazing! This woman was completely unaware of the number of calories all this cake represented. The cake alone must have amounted to roughly 1000 calories per day. So her actual caloric intake was probably more like 2900 per day.

I knew Doris was 37 years old, about 5′ 5″, and probably 190 pounds. Later, I checked the Weight Maintenance Calorie Table on page 140 and found that to maintain 190 pounds at an Activity Level of 2 (she puts in a long day—on her feet most of the time) requires 2881 calories per day. Check! That explained her weight level. My confidence in science was restored!

I returned to the store that evening and convinced Doris that her weight problem could be solved if she went on a sound reducing diet. First, I suggested she have a medical check-up and then that she try my 1200 calorie diet. "Once you reduce," I said, "maintaining your weight should be easy. Just eat as you do now, minus the cake!"

Overseas Assignment

One of my card-playing buddies is a 43-year-old physicist named Carl. Considerably overweight at 5' 9" and 200 pounds, he had decided to start on a reducing diet. His goal was to lose 30 pounds—at 170 pounds he would be at the same weight he was twenty years before, when he graduated from college.

My approach to the subject, and the numerical exactness of the tables, delighted him. He wasn't the most active person I had ever known. (His idea of roughing it was playing pinochle in a room with the window open two inches—from the top.) He didn't quite view himself in this way, however, and it practically took an argument before he would agree to Activity Level 1.

Beyond that point he needed no help. Referring to the Weight Loss Calorie Table that applied to him (page 61), he selected an 1800 calorie diet option. With mathematical precision, Carl lost twenty pounds in eleven weeks, accounting for every pound in a notebook. Then it happened.

He had reluctantly accepted a temporary assignment in France and would be away for six months! One of the card players moaned that he was ruining our card game.

"The hell with the card game," he bellowed, "what about my diet! How am I going to cope with all that French food?"

"Go on maintenance," I replied. "You are at 180 pounds. Try to return at the same weight, and we can pick up the diet right where you left off."

From his Weight Maintenance Calorie Table on page 134, we found he could eat at a 2690 calorie level per day (that represents quite a bit of French food) and still maintain his weight at 180 pounds.

Six months passed, and he returned at 182 pounds. Not bad! Buoyed by his success and becoming impatient, he went on a 1500 calorie diet and reached 170 pounds in approximately 40 days.

Incidentally, although his weight level is now the same as it was twenty years ago, his weight *distribution* is quite different. Carl lost more than 3 inches in his waist measurement, and yet when he tried on the army uniform he had worn at age 23, he found the pants much too tight around the waist (about four inches too tight). Obviously, unless you engage in some very strenuous muscle-building activity, the ratio of fat to muscle must increase with age.

Every-Other-Day

A young salesgirl recently asked me what I thought about an "every-other-day" diet; that is, one day on the diet, the next day off the diet.

"No reason why it shouldn't work," I said. "There are, however, two aspects of that kind of routine that worry me. The first is: because you are on that type of diet quite a bit longer than a more conventional plan, you might be more apt to stray. The second point of concern is: what do you eat every other day? You know you really have to diet the second day too—only at a higher calorie level."

"It might not be so bad in my case. I only want to lose 10 pounds."

That was a good point. "Okay," I replied, "I'll work it out both ways for you."

The girl was 23 years of age, 5' 7" tall, and 130 pounds (Activity Level 2). In order to lose two pounds per week, her diet should last five weeks or approximately 35 days. From the Weight Loss Calorie Table on page 94, I found she could lose ten pounds in 33 days on a 1200 calorie diet.

Now let's look at the problem from the "every-other-day" on a diet viewpoint. The first item to decide is what caloric intake to assign to the day you don't diet. My opinion is that the off-day (when you're not dieting), you should be on maintenance. Using the Weight Maintenance Table on page 142, I calculated that her average maintenance level during a weight reduction from 130 to 120 pounds would be 2350 calories per day.

We agreed that her food intake on off-diet days would be 2350 calories. If she restricted herself to 1200 calories one day, 2350 the next, then 1200, then 2350, and so forth, her average intake over the diet period would be approximately 1800 calories per day. Again referring to the Weight Loss Calorie Table on page 94, but this time using 1800 as the value for the diet calories, we find it would now take 68 days to lose ten pounds.

Motivated by the fact that it was already May 15, and summer (and bikini time) was only a month away, she decided to go straight—a straight 1200 calories per day for 33 days.

POSTSCRIPT

Statistics show that approximately 60,000,000 people in the United States are overweight to some extent. Why? The main culprit is modern technology. The technology that developed chemical fertilizers, insecticides and farm machinery, the automobile, elevator, bulldozer, power tools, dishwasher, and washing machine. In other words, the technology that revolutionized food production and created our modern energy saving devices. We are living in a food-abundant society in which strenuous physical activity is, for most people, a thing of the past. The result is an overweight population.

As a consequence of this and other aspects of modern life, there has been a shift toward an anti-technology point of view—particularly among young people. In their eyes, technological development is all bad. I disagree. I feel that constructive technological innovation, be it in engineering or in the pure sciences, is our main hope for solving many of our physical, social, and environmental problems.

Technology has unquestionably satisfied many human needs and provided enormous benefits to society. But we do have to learn how to cope with much of this progress. We have created a society in which one must be conscious of the amount of food consumed, otherwise too much might be eaten; and in which one must make a real effort to obtain sufficient physical exercise.

The main theme of this book has been that in order to

successfully control your weight you must: be reasonably well informed with regard to the many aspects of weight control; have access to the best data available; know how to use the data to devise a sound weight control plan; and finally, have the fortitude to adhere to your plan.

I admit that the engineer is responsible for much of the modern technology that has made it so tragically easy for so many people to be overweight. It is perhaps fitting that it is an engineer who provides you with the means to erase these previous technological "gains." The use of the modern digital computer to provide the data in this book represents what I deem constructive technology.

It is my hope that you will find it useful.

APPENDIX A
900 CALORIE—7-DAY COMPUTER DIET FOR WOMEN **

	Breakfast (200 calories)	Mid-morning Snack (0 calories)	Lunch (300 calories)	Dinner (400 calories)	Evening Snack (0 calories)
Day 1	4 oz. orange juice Soft boiled egg Toast* Black coffee	Cup of bouillon	3/4 cup cottage cheese 1/2 cup green beans Tea with lemon	4 oz. broiled steak 1/2 baked potato Slice of bread* 4 oz. skim milk Fresh fruit	Green salad lemon and tomato dressing
Day 2	1/2 grapefruit Cup cereal with 5 oz. skim milk Black coffee	Black coffee	4 oz. hamburger 1/2 cup cole slaw Non-caloric soft drink	4 oz. flounder 1/2 cup broccoli 8 oz. skim milk Slice of bread*	Celery and carrot sticks
Day 3	1 cup strawberries Poached egg Toast* Black coffee	Cup of bouillon	4 oz. tuna fish 1/2 cup asparagus Slice of bread* 4 oz. skim milk	4 oz. lamb chop 1/2 cup apple sauce 8 oz. skim milk Plain cookie	Green salad lemon and tomato dressing
Day 4	4 oz. orange juice Soft boiled egg Toast* Black coffee	Black coffee	3/4 cup cottage cheese 1/2 cup green beans Tea with lemon	4 oz. roast beef 1/2 baked potato Slice of bread* 4 oz. skim milk Fresh fruit	Celery and carrot sticks

Day 5	1/2 cantaloupe Cup cereal with 5 oz. skim milk Black coffee	Cup of bouillon	Mushroom omelet Slice of bread* Regular coffee Fresh fruit	4 oz. halibut 1/2 cup kale 8 oz. skim milk Slice of bread*	Green salad lemon and tomato dressing
Day 6	4 oz. pineapple juice Soft boiled egg Toast* Black coffee	Black coffee	4 oz. hamburger Medium tomato Tea with lemon	4 oz. roast chicken 1/2 cup spinach 8 oz. skim milk Fresh fruit	Celery and carrot sticks
Day 7	4 oz. grapefruit juice Poached egg Toast* Black coffee	Cup of bouillon	4 oz. tuna fish 1/2 cup cole slaw Slice of bread* 4 oz. skim milk	4 oz. veal chop 1/2 cup cauliflower 8 oz. skim milk Fresh fruit	Green salad lemon and tomato dressing

Most unsweetened cereals are allowed. Do not add sugar to cereal and use none in black coffee or tea. Regular coffee contains 1 oz. of whole milk and 1 tsp. of sugar. Tuna fish must be water-packed type. Cottage cheese may be creamed variety. Meat must be lean and trimmed of fat. Different meat and fish types may be substituted for those indicated. However, the amounts should not be changed. An unlimited amount of green salad may be eaten; 2 tbsp. salad dressing may be used if so indicated. Where soup is indicated, it must be water-base type. If toast or bread is designated * use no butter; otherwise ½ pat of butter is permitted.
** This diet is intended for younger (pre-menopausal) women.

1200 CALORIE—7-DAY COMPUTER DIET FOR WOMEN ✳︎✳︎

	Breakfast (200 calories)	Mid-morning Snack (0 calories)	Lunch (350 calories)	Dinner (500 calories)	Evening Snack (150 calories)
Day 1	4 oz. orange juice Soft boiled egg Toast* Black coffee	Cup of bouillon	1 cup cottage cheese 1/2 cup green beans Tea with lemon	4 oz. broiled steak 1/2 baked potato Buttered bread 4 oz. skim milk Fresh fruit	Black coffee and small piece of plain cake
Day 2	1/2 grapefruit Cup cereal with 5 oz. skim milk Black coffee	Black coffee	4 oz. hamburger 1/2 cup cole slaw Slice of bread* Non-caloric soft drink	6 oz. flounder 1/2 cup of rice 1/2 cup broccoli 8 oz. skim milk	Cup of flavored gelatin
Day 3	1 cup strawberries Poached egg Toast* Black coffee	Cup of bouillon	4 oz. tuna fish 1/2 cup asparagus Slice of bread* 4 oz. skim milk	4 oz. lamb chops Baked potato 1/2 cup apple sauce Regular coffee Plain cookie	1/2 cup of flavored yogurt
Day 4	4 oz. orange juice Soft boiled egg Toast* Black coffee	Black coffee	1 cup cottage cheese 1/2 cup green beans Tea with lemon	4 oz. roast beef 1/2 baked potato Buttered bread 4 oz. skim milk Fresh fruit	Regular coffee and toast with jam

Day 5	1/2 cantaloupe Cup cereal with 5 oz. skim milk Black coffee	Cup of bouillon	Mushroom omelet Slice of bread* Regular coffee Banana	6 oz. halibut Baked potato 1/2 cup kale 8 oz. skim milk	Cup of flavored gelatin
Day 6	4 oz. pineapple juice Soft boiled egg Toast* Black coffee	Black coffee	4 oz. hamburger Medium tomato Slice of bread* Tea with lemon	6 oz. roast chicken 1/2 cup spinach 4 oz. skim milk Fresh fruit	4 oz. skim milk and 2 graham crackers
Day 7	4 oz. grapefruit juice Poached egg Toast* Black coffee	Cup of bouillon	4 oz. tuna fish 1/2 cup cole slaw Slice of bread* 4 oz. skim milk	4 oz. veal chops 1/2 cup of rice 1/2 cup cauliflower Regular coffee Fresh fruit	1/2 cup of ice cream

Most unsweetened cereals are allowed. Do not add sugar to cereal and use none in black coffee or tea. Regular coffee contains 1 oz. of whole milk and 1 tsp. of sugar. Tuna fish may be oil-packed type, well drained. Cottage cheese may be creamed variety. Meat must be lean and trimmed of fat. Different meat and fish types may be substituted for those indicated. However, the amounts should not be changed. An unlimited amount of green salad may be eaten; 2 tbsp. salad dressing may be used if so indicated. Where soup is indicated, it must be a water-base type. If toast or bread is designated * use no butter; otherwise ½ pat of butter is permitted.

** This diet is intended for younger (pre-menopausal) women.

1500 CALORIE—7-DAY COMPUTER DIET FOR WOMEN * *

	Breakfast (250 calories)	Mid-morning Snack (0 calories)	Lunch (450 calories)	Dinner (650 calories)	Evening Snack (150 calories)
Day 1	4 oz. orange juice Soft boiled egg Buttered toast Regular coffee	Cup of bouillon	1 cup cottage cheese 1/2 cup green beans Banana Regular tea	6 oz. broiled steak Baked potato Buttered bread 4 oz. skim milk Fresh fruit	Black coffee and small piece of plain cake
Day 2	1/2 grapefruit Cup of cereal with 5 oz. skim milk Regular coffee	Black coffee	4 oz. hamburger 1/2 cup cole slaw Buttered bread Non-caloric soft drink Fresh fruit	6 oz. flounder Cup of rice 1/2 cup broccoli 8 oz. skim milk	Cup of flavored gelatin
Day 3	1 cup strawberries Poached egg Buttered toast Regular coffee	Cup of bouillon	6 oz. tuna fish 1/2 cup asparagus Slice of bread* 4 oz. skim milk	6 oz. lamb chops Baked potato 1/2 cup apple sauce Regular coffee Plain cookie	1/2 cup of flavored yogurt
Day 4	4 oz. orange juice Soft boiled egg Buttered toast Regular coffee	Black coffee	1 cup cottage cheese 1/2 cup green beans Tomato Regular tea	6 oz. roast beef Baked potato Buttered bread 4 oz. skim milk Fresh fruit	Regular coffee and toast with jam

Day 5	1/2 cantaloupe Cup of cereal with 5 oz. skim milk Regular coffee	Cup of bouillon	Cup of soup Mushroom omelet Slice of bread* Regular coffee Banana	6 oz. halibut Baked potato 1/2 cup kale Slice of bread* 8 oz. skim milk	Cup of flavored gelatin
Day 6	4 oz. pineapple juice Soft boiled egg Buttered toast Regular coffee	Black coffee	4 oz. hamburger Tomato Cucumber salad Buttered bread Tea with lemon	6 oz. roast chicken 1/2 cup spinach 8 oz. skim milk Fresh fruit	4 oz. skim milk and 2 graham crackers
Day 7	4 oz. grapefruit juice Poached egg Buttered toast Regular coffee	Cup of bouillon	6 oz. tuna fish 1/2 cup cole slaw Slice of bread* 4 oz. skim milk	6 oz. veal chops 1/2 cup of rice 1/2 cup cauliflower Regular coffee Fresh fruit	1/2 cup of ice cream

Most unsweetened cereals are allowed. Do not add sugar to cereal and use none in black coffee or tea. Regular coffee contains 1 oz. of whole milk and 1 tsp. of sugar. Tuna fish may be oil-packed type, well drained. Cottage cheese may be creamed variety. Meat must be lean and trimmed of fat. Different meat and fish types may be substituted for those indicated. However, the amounts should not be changed. An unlimited amount of green salad may be eaten; 2 tbsp. salad dressing may be used if so indicated. Where soup is indicated, it must be a water-base type. If toast or bread is designated * use no butter; otherwise 1/2 pat of butter is permitted.

** This diet is intended for younger (pre-menopausal) women.

1800 CALORIE—7-DAY COMPUTER DIET FOR WOMEN * *

	Breakfast (400 calories)	Mid-morning Snack (50 calories)	Lunch (450 calories)	Dinner (750 calories)	Evening Snack (150 calories)
Day 1	4 oz. orange juice Fried egg 2 strips bacon Buttered toast Regular coffee	Fresh fruit	1 cup cottage cheese 1/2 cup green beans Banana Regular tea	8 oz. broiled steak Baked potato Slice of bread* 4 oz. skim milk Fresh fruit	Black coffee and small piece of plain cake
Day 2	1/2 grapefruit Cereal with milk Soft boiled egg Toast* Regular coffee	Black coffee or tea and a plain cookie	4 oz. hamburger 1/2 cup cole slaw Buttered bread Non-caloric soft drink Fresh fruit	8 oz. flounder Cup of rice 1/2 cup broccoli Slice of bread* 8 oz. skim milk	Cup of flavored gelatin
Day 3	1 cup strawberries 1 pancake 2 strips bacon 2 tbsp. syrup Regular coffee	Black coffee or tea and 3 soda crackers	6 oz. tuna fish 1/2 cup asparagus Slice of bread* 4 oz. skim milk	6 oz. lamb chops Baked potato 1/2 cup apple sauce Buttered bread Regular coffee Fresh fruit	1/2 cup of flavored yogurt
Day 4	4 oz. orange juice Poached egg 2 strips bacon Buttered toast Regular coffee	Fresh fruit	1 cup cottage cheese 1/2 cup green beans Tomato Regular tea	8 oz. roast beef Baked potato Slice of bread* 4 oz. skim milk Fresh fruit	Regular coffee and toast with jam

Day					
Day 5	1/2 cantaloupe Cereal with milk Soft boiled egg Toast* Regular coffee	Black coffee or tea and a plain cookie	Cup of soup Mushroom omelet Slice of bread* Regular coffee Banana	8 oz. halibut Baked potato 1/2 cup kale Buttered bread 8 oz. skim milk Fresh fruit	Cup of flavored gelatin
Day 6	4 oz. pineapple juice 1 French toast 2 strips bacon 2 tbsp. syrup Regular coffee	4 oz. skim milk	4 oz. hamburger Tomato Cucumber salad Buttered bread Tea with lemon	8 oz. roast chicken Baked potato 1/2 cup spinach 4 oz. skim milk Fresh fruit	Regular coffee and 2 graham crackers
Day 7	4 oz. grapefruit juice Fried egg 2 strips of bacon Buttered toast Regular coffee	Fresh fruit	6 oz. tuna fish 1/2 cup cole slaw Slice of bread* 4 oz. skim milk	8 oz. veal chops 1/2 cup of rice 1/2 cup cauliflower Non-caloric soft drink Fresh fruit	1/2 cup of ice cream

Most unsweetened cereals are allowed. Do not add sugar to cereal and use none in black coffee or tea. Regular coffee contains 1 oz. of whole milk and 1 tsp. of sugar. Tuna fish may be oil-packed type, well drained. Cottage cheese may be creamed variety. Meat must be lean and trimmed of fat. Different meat and fish types may be substituted for those indicated. However, the amounts should not be changed. An unlimited amount of green salad may be eaten; 2 tbsp. salad dressing may be used if so indicated. Where soup is indicated, it must be a water-base type. If toast or bread is designated * use no butter; otherwise ½ pat of butter is permitted.

** This diet is intended for younger (pre-menopausal) women.

900 CALORIE—7 DAY COMPUTER DIET FOR MEN * *

	Breakfast (200 calories)	Mid-morning Snack (0 calories)	Lunch (300 calories)	Dinner (400 calories)	Evening Snack (0 calories)
Day 1	4 oz. orange juice Soft-boiled egg Toast* Black coffee	Cup of bouillon	3/4 cup cottage cheese 1/2 cup green beans Tea with lemon	4 oz. broiled steak 1/2 baked potato Slice of bread* 4 oz. skim milk Fresh fruit	Green salad lemon and tomato dressing
Day 2	1/2 grapefruit Cup cereal with 5 oz. skim milk Black coffee	Black coffee	4 oz. hamburger 1/2 cup cole slaw Non-caloric soda	4 oz. flounder 1/2 cup broccoli 8 oz. skim milk Slice of bread*	Celery and carrot sticks
Day 3	Strawberries (1 cup) Cup cereal with 5 oz. skim milk Black coffee	Cup of bouillon	4 oz. tuna fish 1/2 cup asparagus Slice of bread* 4 oz. skim milk	4 oz. lamb chop 1/2 cup apple sauce Regular coffee Plain cookie	Green salad lemon and tomato dressing
Day 4	4 oz. orange juice Cup cereal with 5 oz. skim milk Black coffee	Black coffee	3/4 cup cottage cheese 1/2 cup green beans Tea with lemon	4 oz. roast beef 1/2 baked potato Slice of bread* 4 oz. skim milk Fresh fruit	Celery and carrot sticks

Day 5	1/2 cantaloupe Cup cereal with 5 oz. skim milk Black coffee	Cup of bouillon	4 oz. turkey 1/2 cup cole slaw Slice of bread Fresh fruit	4 oz. halibut 1/2 cup kale 8 oz. skim milk Slice of bread* Green salad lemon and tomato dressing
Day 6	4 oz. pineapple juice Poached egg Toast* Black coffee	Black coffee	4 oz. hamburger Medium tomato Tea with lemon	4 oz. roast chicken 1/2 cup spinach 8 oz. skim milk Fresh fruit Celery and carrot sticks
Day 7	4 oz. grapefruit juice Cup cereal with 5 oz. skim milk Black coffee	Cup of bouillon	4 oz. tuna fish 1/2 cup cole slaw Slice of bread* 4 oz. skim milk	4 oz. veal chop 1/2 cup cauliflower Regular coffee Fresh fruit Green salad lemon and tomato dressing

Most unsweetened cereals are allowed. Do not add sugar to cereal and use none in black coffee or tea. Regular coffee contains 1 oz. of whole milk and 1 tsp. of sugar. Tuna fish must be water-packed type. Cottage cheese may be creamed variety. Meat must be lean and trimmed of fat. Different meat and fish types may be substituted for those indicated. However, the amounts should not be changed. An unlimited amount of green salad may be eaten; 2 tbsp. salad dressing may be used if so indicated. Where soup is indicated, it must be a water-base type. If toast or bread is designated * use no spread, otherwise ½ pat of margarine or ½ tsp. of jelly is permitted.

** This diet is also recommended for women past menopause.

1200 CALORIE—7 DAY COMPUTER DIET FOR MEN **

	Breakfast (200 calories)	Mid-morning Snack (0 calories)	Lunch (350 calories)	Dinner (500 calories)	Evening Snack (150 calories)
Day 1	4 oz. orange juice Soft boiled egg Toast* Black coffee	Cup of bouillon	1 cup cottage cheese 1/2 cup green beans Tea with lemon	4 oz. broiled steak 1/2 baked potato 4 oz. skim milk Fresh fruit	Black coffee and small piece of plain cake
Day 2	1/2 grapefruit Cup cereal with 5 oz. skim milk Black coffee	Black coffee	4 oz. hamburger 1/2 cup cole slaw Slice of bread* Non-caloric soda	6 oz. flounder Cup of rice 1/2 cup broccoli 8 oz. skim milk	Cup of flavored gelatin
Day 3	Strawberries (1 cup) Cup cereal with 5 oz. skim milk Black coffee	Cup of bouillon	4 oz. tuna fish 1/2 cup asparagus Slice of bread* 4 oz. skim milk	4 oz. lamb chops Baked potato 1/2 cup apple sauce Regular coffee Plain cookie	1/2 cup of flavored yogurt
Day 4	4 oz. orange juice Cup cereal with 5 oz. skim milk Black coffee	Black coffee	1 cup cottage cheese 1/2 cup green beans Tea with lemon	4 oz. roast beef 1/2 baked potato Slice of bread* 4 oz. skim milk Fresh fruit	Regular coffee and toast with jam

Day 5	1/2 cantaloupe Cup cereal with 5 oz. skim milk Black coffee	Cup of bouillon	4 oz. turkey 1/2 cup cole slaw Slice of bread Fresh fruit	6 oz. halibut Baked potato 1/2 cup kale 8 oz. skim milk	Cup of flavored gelatin
Day 6	4 oz. pineapple juice Poached egg Toast* Black coffee	Black coffee	4 oz. hamburger Medium tomato Slice of bread Tea with lemon	6 oz. roast chicken 1/2 cup spinach 4 oz. skim milk Fresh fruit	4 oz. skim milk and 2 graham crackers
Day 7	4 oz. grapefruit juice Cup cereal with 5 oz. skim milk Black coffee	Cup of bouillon	4 oz. tuna fish 1/2 cup cole slaw Slice of bread* 4 oz. skim milk	4 oz. veal chop Cup of rice 1/2 cup cauliflower Regular coffee Fresh fruit	1/2 cup of sherbet

Most unsweetened cereals are allowed. Do not add sugar to cereal and use none in black coffee or tea. Regular coffee contains 1 oz. of whole milk and 1 tsp. of sugar. Tuna fish must be water-packed type. Cottage cheese may be creamed variety. Meat must be lean and trimmed of fat. Different meat and fish types may be substituted for those indicated. However, the amounts should not be changed. An unlimited amount of green salad may be eaten; 2 tbsp. salad dressing may be used if so indicated. Where soup is indicated, it must be a water-base type. If toast is designated * use no spread, otherwise ½ pat of margarine or ½ tsp. of jelly is permitted.

** This diet is also recommended for women past menopause.

1500 CALORIE—7 DAY COMPUTER DIET FOR MEN **

	Breakfast (250 calories)	Mid-morning Snack (0 calories)	Lunch (450 calories)	Dinner (650 calories)	Evening Snack (150 calories)
Day 1	4 oz. orange juice Soft boiled egg Toast* Regular coffee	Cup of bouillon	1 cup cottage cheese 1/2 cup green beans Banana Regular tea	6 oz. broiled steak Baked potato Slice of bread* 4 oz. skim milk Fresh fruit	Black coffee and small piece of plain cake
Day 2	1/2 grapefruit Cup of cereal with 5 oz. skim milk Regular coffee	Black coffee	4 oz. hamburger 1/2 cup cole slaw Slice of bread* Non-caloric soda Fresh fruit	6 oz. flounder Cup of rice 1/2 cup broccoli 8 oz. skim milk	Cup of flavored gelatin
Day 3	Strawberries (1 cup) Cup of cereal with 5 oz. skim milk Regular coffee	Cup of bouillon	6 oz. tuna fish 1/2 cup asparagus Slice of bread 4 oz. skim milk	6 oz. lamb chops Baked potato 1/2 cup apple sauce Regular coffee Plain cookie	1/2 cup of flavored yogurt
Day 4	4 oz. orange juice Cup of cereal with 5 oz. skim milk Regular coffee	Black coffee	1 cup cottage cheese 1/2 cup green beans Tomato Regular tea Slice of bread	6 oz. roast beef Baked potato Slice of bread* 4 oz. skim milk Fresh fruit	Regular coffee and toast with jam

Day 5	1/2 cantaloupe Cup of cereal with 5 oz. skim milk Regular coffee	Cup of bouillon	6 oz. turkey 1/2 cup cole slaw Slice of bread* Fresh fruit	6 oz. halibut Baked potato 1/2 cup kale Slice of bread* 8 oz. skim milk	Cup of flavored gelatin
Day 6	4 oz. pineapple juice Poached egg Toast* Regular coffee	Black coffee	4 oz. hamburger Tomato Cucumber salad Slice of bread* Tea with lemon	6 oz. roast chicken 1/2 cup spinach 8 oz. skim milk Fresh fruit	4 oz. skim milk and 2 graham crackers
Day 7	4 oz. grapefruit juice Cup of cereal with 5 oz. skim milk Regular coffee	Cup of bouillon	6 oz. tuna fish 1/2 cup cole slaw Slice of bread 4 oz. skim milk	6 oz. veal chops Cup of rice 1/2 cup cauliflower Regular coffee Fresh fruit	1/2 cup of sherbet

Most unsweetened cereals are allowed. Do no add sugar to cereal and use none in black coffee or tea. Regular coffee contains 1 oz. of whole milk and 1 tsp. of sugar. Tuna fish must be water-packed type. Cottage cheese may be creamed variety. Meat must be lean and trimmed of fat. Different meat and fish types may be substituted for those indicated. However, the amounts should not be changed. An unlimited amount of green salad may be eaten; 2 tbsp. salad dressing may be used if so indicated. Where soup is indicated, it must be a water-base type. If toast or bread is designated * use no spread, otherwise ½ pat of margarine or ½ tsp. of jelly is permitted.
** This diet is also recommended for women past menopause.

1800 CALORIE—7 DAY COMPUTER DIET FOR MEN *

	Breakfast (400 calories)	Mid-morning Snack (50 calories)	Lunch (450 calories)	Dinner (750 calories)	Evening Snack (150 calories)
Day 1	4 oz. orange juice Cereal with milk Toast Regular coffee	Fresh fruit in season	1 cup cottage cheese 1/2 cup green beans Banana Regular tea	8 oz. broiled steak Baked potato Slice of bread 4 oz. skim milk Fruit in season	Black coffee and small piece of plain cake
Day 2	1/2 grapefruit Cereal with milk Soft boiled egg Toast* Regular coffee	Black coffee or tea and a plain cookie	4 oz. hamburger 1/2 cup cole slaw Slice of bread* Non-caloric soda Fresh fruit	8 oz. flounder Cup of rice 1/2 cup broccoli Slice of bread* 8 oz. skim milk	Cup of flavored gelatin
Day 3	Strawberries (1 cup) Cereal with milk Toast Regular coffee	Black coffee or tea and 3 soda crackers	6 oz. tuna fish 1/2 cup asparagus Slice of bread* 4 oz. skim milk	6 oz. lamb chops Baked potato 1/2 cup apple sauce Slice of bread Regular coffee Fresh fruit	1/2 cup of flavored yogurt
Day 4	4 oz. orange juice Cereal with milk Toast Regular coffee	Fresh fruit in season	1 cup cottage cheese 1/2 cup green beans Tomato Regular tea	8 oz. roast beef Baked potato Slice of bread* 4 oz. skim milk Fruit in season	Regular coffee and toast with jam

Day 5	1/2 cantaloupe Cereal with milk Toast Regular coffee	Black coffee or tea and a plain cookie	6 oz. turkey 1/2 cup cole slaw Slice of bread Fresh fruit	8 oz. halibut Baked potato 1/2 cup kale Slice of bread* 8 oz. skim milk Fresh fruit	Cup of flavored gelatin
Day 6	4 oz. pineapple juice Cereal with milk Poached egg Toast* Regular coffee	4 oz. skim milk	4 oz. hamburger Tomato Cucumber salad Slice of bread* Tea with lemon	8 oz. roast chicken Baked potato 1/2 cup spinach 4 oz. skim milk Fresh fruit	Regular coffee and 2 graham crackers
Day 7	4 oz. grapefruit juice Cereal with milk Toast Regular coffee	Fresh fruit in season	6 oz. tuna fish 1/2 cup cole slaw Slice of bread 4 oz. skim milk	8 oz. veal chops Cup of rice 1/2 cup cauliflower Non-caloric soda Fresh fruit	1/2 cup of sherbet

Most unsweetened cereals are allowed. Do not add sugar to cereal and use none in black coffee or tea. Regular coffee contains 1 oz. of whole milk and 1 tsp. of sugar. Tuna fish must be water-packed type. Cottage cheese may be creamed variety. Meat must be lean and trimmed of fat. Different meat and fish types may be substituted for those indicated. However, the amounts should not be changed. An unlimited amount of green salad may be eaten; 2 tbsp. salad dressing may be **used** if so indicated. Where soup is indicated, it must be a water-base type. If **toast** or **bread** is designated * use no spread, otherwise ½ pat of margarine or ½ tsp. of jelly is permitted.

** This diet is also recommended for women past menopause.

2100 CALORIE—7-DAY COMPUTER DIET FOR MEN

	Breakfast (500 calories)	Mid-morning Snack (50 calories)	Lunch (450 calories)	Dinner (950 calories)	Evening Snack (150 calories)
Day 1	4 oz. orange juice Cereal with milk and fresh fruit Toast Regular coffee	Black coffee or tea and 3 soda crackers	1 cup cottage cheese 1/2 cup green beans Banana Regular tea	8 oz. broiled steak Baked potato 2 tbsp. salad oil Slice of bread* 8 oz. skim milk Fruit in season	Black coffee and small piece of plain cake
Day 2	1/2 grapefruit Cereal with milk 1 soft boiled egg 2 strips bacon Toast Regular coffee	Fresh fruit	4 oz. hamburger 1/2 cup cole slaw Slice of bread Non-caloric soft drink Fresh fruit	8 oz. flounder Cup of rice 1/2 cup broccoli 2 tbsp. salad oil Slice of bread* 8 oz. skim milk	Cup of flavored gelatin
Day 3	4 oz. grapefruit juice Cereal with milk and fresh fruit Toast Regular coffee	Fresh fruit	6 oz. tuna fish 1/2 cup asparagus Slice of bread 8 oz. skim milk	Cup of soup 8 oz. lamb chops Baked potato 1/2 cup apple sauce Slice of bread Regular coffee	1/2 cup of flavored yogurt
Day 4	4 oz. orange juice Cereal with milk and fresh fruit Toast Regular coffee	Fresh fruit	1 cup cottage cheese 1/2 cup green beans Tomato Regular tea	8 oz. roast beef Baked potato Slice of bread 8 oz. skim milk Fruit in season	Regular coffee and toast with jam

Day 5	4 oz. pineapple juice Cereal with milk and fresh fruit Toast Regular coffee	Black coffee or tea and a plain cookie	6 oz. turkey 1/2 cup cole slaw Slice of bread* Fresh fruit	8 oz. halibut Baked potato 1/2 cup kale 2 tbsp. salad oil Slice of bread 8 oz. skim milk	Cup of flavored gelatin
Day 6	1/2 cantaloupe Cereal with milk Soft-boiled egg 2 strips bacon Toast Regular coffee	4 oz. skim milk	4 oz. hamburger Tomato Cucumber salad Slice of bread Tea with lemon	8 oz. roast chicken Baked potato 2 tbsp. salad oil 1/2 cup spinach 8 oz. skim milk Fresh fruit	Regular coffee and 2 graham crackers
Day 7	4 oz. grapefruit juice Cereal with milk and fresh fruit Toast Regular coffee	Fresh fruit	6 oz. tuna fish 1/2 cup cole slaw Slice of bread* 8 oz. skim milk	Cup of soup 8 oz. veal chops 1/2 cup of rice 1/2 cup cauliflower Regular coffee Fresh fruit	Cup of sherbet

Most unsweetened cereals are allowed. Do not add sugar to cereal and use none in black coffee or tea. Regular coffee contains 1 oz. of whole milk and 1 tsp. of sugar. Tuna fish must be water-packed type. Cottage cheese may be creamed variety. Meat must be lean and trimmed of fat. Different meat and fish types may be substituted for those indicated. However, the amounts should not be changed. An unlimited amount of green salad may be eaten; 2 tbsp. salad dressing may be used if so indicated. Where soup is indicated, it must be a water-base type. If toast or bread is designated * use no spread, otherwise ½ pat of margarine or ½ tsp. of jelly is permitted.

APPENDIX B
CALORIC VALUE OF SELECTED FOODS

MEAT, POULTRY, FISH, EGGS, DRY BEANS AND PEAS, NUTS

		Number of calories
Meat, cooked, without bone:		
Beef:		
Pot roast or braised:		
Lean and fat	3 ounces (1 thick or 2 thin slices, 4 × 2½ inches).	245
Lean only	2½ ounces (1 thick or 2 thin slices, 4 × 2 inches).	140
Oven roast:		
Cut having relatively large proportion of fat to lean:		
Lean and fat	3 ounces (1 thick or 2 thin slices, 4 × 2½ inches).	375
Lean only	2 ounces (1 thick or 2 thin slices, 4 × 1½ inches).	140
Cut having relatively low proportion of fat to lean:		
Lean and fat	3 ounces (1 thick or 2 thin slices, 4 × 2½ inches).	165
Lean only	2½ ounces (1 thick or 2 thin slices, 4 × 2 inches).	115
Steak, broiled:		
Lean and fat	3 ounces (1 piece, 4 × 2½ inches × ½ inch).	330
Lean only	2 ounces (1 piece, 4 × 1½ inches × ½ inch).	115

(Adapted from U.S. Department of Agriculture Home and Garden Bulletin No. 74)

Caloric Value of Selected Foods

MEAT, POULTRY, FISH, EGGS, DRY BEANS AND PEAS, NUTS—Continued

		Number of calories
Hamburger patty:		
Regular ground beef..	3-ounce patty (about 4 patties per pound of raw meat).	245
Lean ground round ...	3-ounce patty (about 4 patties per pound of raw meat).	185
Corned beef, canned	3 ounces (1 piece, 4 × 2½ inches × ½ inch).	185
Corned beef hash, canned	3 ounces (scant half cup)	155
Dried beef, chipped	2 ounces (about ⅓ cup) ..	115
Meat loaf	2 ounces (1 piece, 4 × 2½ inches × ½ inch).	115
Beef and vegetable stew	½ cup	105
Beef pot pie, baked	1 pie (4¼ inch diameter, about 8 ounces before baking).	560
Chile con carne, canned:		
Without beans	½ cup	255
With beans	½ cup	170
Veal:		
Cutlet, broiled, meat only	3 ounces (1 piece, 4 × 2½ inches × ½ inch).	185
Lamb:		
Chop (about 2½ chops to a pound, as purchased):		
Lean and fat	4 ounces	400
Lean only	2¾ ounces	140
Roast, leg:		
Lean and fat	3 ounces (1 thick or 2 thin slices, 3½ × 3 inches).	235
Lean only	2½ ounces (1 thick or 2 thin slices, 3½ × 2½ inches).	130
Pork:		
Fresh:		
Chop (about 3 chops to a pound, as purchased):		
Lean and fat	2⅓ ounces	260
Lean only	2 ounces	155
Roast, loin:		

MEAT, POULTRY, FISH, EGGS, DRY BEANS AND PEAS, NUTS—Continued

		Number of calories
Lean and fat	3 ounces (1 thick or 2 thin slices, 4 × 2½ inches).	310
Lean only	2⅔ ounces (1 thick or 2 thin slices, 3 × 2½ inches).	175
Cured: Ham:		
Lean and fat	3 ounces (1 thick or 2 thin slices, 4 × 2 inches).	245
Lean only	2⅛ ounces (1 thick or 2 thin slices, 3½ × 2 inches).	120
Bacon, broiled or fried	2 very thin strips	100
Sausage, variety, and luncheon meats:		
Bologna sausage	2 ounces (2 very thin slices, 4 inches in diameter).	170
Liver sausage (liverwurst)	2 ounces (4 very thin slices, 3 inches in diameter).	175
Vienna sausage, canned	2 ounces (4 to 5 sausages).	135
Pork sausage, bulk	2 ounces (1 patty, 2 inches in diameter), (4 to 5 patties per pound, raw).	270
Liver, beef, fried (includes fat for frying).	2 ounces (1 thick piece, 3 × 2½ inches).	130
Heart, beef, braised, trimmed of fat.	3 ounces (1 thick piece, 4 × 2½ inches).	160
Tongue, beef, braised	3 ounces (1 thick slice, 4 × 2½ inches).	210 155
Frankfurter	1 frankfurter	155
Boiled ham (luncheon meat).	2 ounces (2 very thin slices, 3½ × 3½ inches).	135
Spiced ham, canned	2 ounces (2 thin slices, 3 × 2½ inches).	165
Poultry, cooked, without bone: Chicken:		
Broiled	3 ounces (about ¼ of a small broiler).	185
Fried	½ breast (2⅜ ounces)	155
	1 leg (thigh and drumstick), 3 ounces.	225
Canned	3½ ounces (½ cup)	200

Caloric Value of Selected Foods

MEAT, POULTRY, FISH, EGGS, DRY BEANS AND PEAS, NUTS—Continued

		Number of calories
Poultry pie (with potatoes, peas, and gravy).	1 small pie, 4¼ inches in diameter (about 8 ounces before cooking).	535
Fish and shellfish:		
Bluefish, baked	3 ounces (1 piece, 3½ × 2 inches × ½ inch).	135
Clams, shelled:		
Raw, meat only	3 ounces (about 4 medium clams).	65
Canned, clams and juice.	3 ounces (1 scant half cup, 3 medium clams and juice).	45
Crab meat, canned or cooked.	3 ounces, ½ cup	85
Fish sticks, breaded, cooked, frozen (including breading and fat for frying).	4 ounces (5 fish sticks)	200
Haddock, fried (including fat for frying).	3 ounces (1 fillet, 4 × 2½ inches × ½ inch).	140
Mackerel:		
Broiled	3 ounces (1 piece, 4 × 3 inches × ½ inch).	200
Canned	3 ounces, solids and liquid (about ⅜ cup).	155
Ocean perch, fried (including egg, breadcrumbs, and fat for frying).	3 ounces (1 piece, 4 × 2½ inches × ½ inch).	195
Oysters, shucked: Raw, meat only.	½ cup (6 to 10 medium-size oysters, selects).	80
Salmon:		
Broiled or baked	4 ounces (1 steak, 4½ × 2½ inches × ½ inch).	205
Canned (pink)	3 ounces, solids and liquid, (about ⅜ cup).	120
Sardines, canned in oil	3 ounces, drained solids (5 to 7 medium sardines).	175
Shrimp, canned, meat only.	3 ounces (about 17 medium shrimp).	100
Tunafish, canned in oil, meat only.	3 ounces (about ⅜ cup)	170

MEAT, POULTRY, FISH, EGGS, DRY BEANS AND PEAS, NUTS—Continued

Food	Amount	Number of calories
Eggs:		
Fried (including fat for frying).	1 large egg	100
Hard or soft boiled	1 large egg	80
Scrambled or omelet (including milk and fat for cooking).	1 large egg	110
Poached	1 large egg	80
Dry beans and peas:		
Red kidney beans, canned or cooked.	½ cup, solids and liquid	115
Lima, cooked	½ cup, solids and liquid	130
Baked beans, with tomato or molasses:		
With pork	½ cup	160
Without pork	½ cup	155
Nuts:		
Almonds, shelled	2 tablespoons (about 13 to 15 almonds).	105
Brazil nuts, shelled, broken pieces.	2 tablespoons	115
Cashew nuts, roasted	2 tablespoons (about 4 to 5 nuts).	95
Coconut:		
Fresh, shredded meat	2 tablespoons	40
Dried, shredded, sweetened.	2 tablespoons	45
Peanuts, roasted, shelled	2 tablespoons	105
Peanut butter	1 tablespoon	95
Pecans, shelled halves	2 tablespoons (about 12 to 14 halves).	95
Walnuts, shelled:		
Black or native, chopped	2 tablespoons	100
English or Persian, halves	2 tablespoons (about 7 to 12 halves).	80

MILK, CHEESE, AND ICE CREAM

Food	Amount	Number of calories
Fluid milk:		
Whole	1 cup or glass	160
Skim (fresh or nonfat dry reconstituted).	1 cup or glass	90

MILK, CHEESE, AND ICE CREAM—Continued

Number of calories

Buttermilk	1 cup or glass	90
Evaporated (undiluted)	½ cup	170
Condensed, sweetened (undiluted).	½ cup	490
Half-and-half (milk and cream).	1 cup	325
	1 tablespoon	20
Cream, light	1 tablespoon	30
Cream, heavy whipping	1 tablespoon	55
Yogurt (made from partially skimmed milk).	1 cup	120
Cheese:		
American, Cheddar-type	1 ounce	115
	1-inch cube (¾ ounce)	70
	½ cup, grated (2 ounces)	225
Process American, Cheddar-type.	1 ounce	105
Blue-mold (or Roquefort-type).	1 ounce	105
Cottage, not creamed	2 tablespoons (1 ounce)	25
Cottage, creamed	2 tablespoons (1 ounce)	30
Cream	2 tablespoons (1 ounce)	105
Parmesan, dry, grated	2 tablespoons (⅓ ounce)	40
Swiss	1 ounce	105
Milk beverages:		
Cocoa (all milk)	1 cup	235
Chocolate-flavored milk drink.	1 cup	190
Malted milk	1 cup	280
Chocolate milkshake	One 12-ounce container	520
Ice cream, plain	1 container (3½ fluid ounces)	130
Ice milk	½ cup (4 fluid ounces)	140
Ice cream soda, chocolate	1 large glass	455

VEGETABLES AND FRUITS

Vegetables:		
Asparagus, cooked or canned	6 medium spears or ½ cup cut spears.	20
Beans:		
Lima, green cooked or canned.	½ cup	80

VEGETABLES AND FRUITS—Continued

		Number of calories
Snap, green, wax or yellow, cooked or canned.	½ cup	15
Beets, cooked or canned	½ cup, diced	30
Beet greens, cooked	½ cup	15
Broccoli, cooked	½ cup flower stalks	20
Brussels sprouts, cooked	½ cup	20
Cabbage:		
Raw	½ cup, shredded	10
	1 wedge, 3½ × 4½ inches	25
Cole slaw (with mayonnaise-type salad dressing).	½ cup	60
Cooked	½ cup	20
Carrots:		
Raw	1 carrot, 5½ inches × 1 inch in diameter, or 25 thin slices.	20
	½ cup, grated	20
Cooked	½ cup, diced	20
Cauliflower, cooked	½ cup flower buds	10
Celery, raw	2 large stalks (8 inches long) or 3 small stalks (5 inches long).	10
Chard, cooked	½ cup	15
Collards, cooked	½ cup	30
Corn:		
On cob, cooked	1 ear, 5 inches long	70
Kernels, cooked or canned	½ cup	85
Cress, garden, cooked	½ cup	20
Cucumbers, raw, pared	6 slices, ⅛ in thick, center section.	5
Kale, cooked	½ cup	15
Kohlrabi, cooked	½ cup	20
Lettuce, raw	2 large or 4 small leaves	10
Mushrooms, canned	½ cup	20
Mustard greens, cooked	½ cup	20
Okra, cooked	4 pods (3 inches long, ⅝ inch in diameter).	10
Onions:		
Young, green, raw	6 small, without tops	20

VEGETABLES AND FRUITS—Continued

		Number of calories
Mature:		
Raw	1 onion (2½ inches in diameter).	40
	1 tablespoon, chopped	5
Cooked	½ cup	30
Parsnips, cooked	½ cup	50
Peas, green:		
Cooked or canned	½ cup	60
Peppers, green:		
Raw or cooked	1 medium	10
Potatoes:		
Baked	1 medium, 2½ inches in diameter (5 ounces raw).	90
Boiled	½ cup, diced	50
Chips (including fat for frying).	10 medium (2 inches in diameter).	115
French-fried (including fat for frying):		
Ready-to-eat	10 pieces, 2 inches × ½ inch × ½ inch.	155
Frozen, heated, ready-to-serve.	10 pieces, 2 inches × ½ inch × ½ inch.	125
Hash-browned	½ cup	225
Mashed:		
Milk added	½ cup	60
Milk and fat added	½ cup	90
Pan-fried, beginning with raw potatoes.	½ cup	230
Radishes, raw	4 small	5
Sauerkraut, canned	½ cup	20
Spinach, cooked or canned	½ cup	20
Squash:		
Summer, cooked	½ cup	15
Winter, baked, mashed	½ cup	65
Sweet potatoes:		
Baked in jacket	1 medium, 5 × 2 inches (6 ounces raw).	155
Canned, vacuum or solid pack.	½ cup	120
Tomatoes:		
Raw	1 medium, 2 × 2½ inches (about ⅓ pound).	35

VEGETABLES AND FRUITS—Continued

		Number of calories
Cooked or canned	½ cup	25
Tomato juice, canned	½ cup	20
Turnips, cooked	½ cup	20
Turnip greens, cooked	½ cup	15
Fruits:		
Apples, raw	1 medium, 2½ inches in diameter (about ⅓ pound).	70
Apple juice, canned	½ cup	60
Apple sauce:		
Sweetened	½ cup	115
Unsweetened	½ cup	50
Apricots:		
Raw	3 (about 12 to a pound, as purchased).	55
Canned:		
Water pack	½ cup, halves and liquid	45
Heavy syrup pack	½ cup, halves and syrup	110
Dried, cooked, unsweetened.	½ cup, fruit and juice	120
Frozen, sweetened	½ cup	125
Avocados:		
California varieties	½ of a 10-ounce avocado (3⅓ × 4¼ inches).	185
Florida varieties	½ of a 13-ounce avocado (4 × 3 inches).	160
Bananas, raw	1 banana (6 × 1½ inches, about ⅓ pound).	85
Berries:		
Blackberries, raw	½ cup	40
Blueberries, raw	½ cup	40
Raspberries:		
Fresh, red, raw	½ cup	35
Frozen, red, sweetened	½ cup	120
Fresh, black, raw	½ cup	50
Strawberries:		
Fresh, raw	½ cup	30
Frozen, sweetened	½ cup, sliced	140
Cantaloupe, raw	½ melon, 5 inches in diameter	60
Cherries:		
Raw:		
Sour	½ cup	30

VEGETABLES AND FRUITS—Continued

Number of calories

Sweet, ½ cup		40
Cranberry sauce, canned, sweetened, 1 tablespoon		25
Cranberry juice cocktail, canned, ½ cup		80
Dates, "fresh" and dried, pitted, cut, ½ cup		245
Figs:		
Raw, 3 small (1½ inches in diameter, about ¼ pound)		90
Canned, heavy syrup, ½ cup		110
Dried, 1 large (2 inches × 1 inch)		60
Fruit cocktail, canned in heavy syrup, ½ cup		100
Grapefruit:		
Raw:		
White, ½ medium (4¼ inches in diameter)		55
½ cup sections		40
Pink or red, ½ medium (4¼ inches in diameter)		60
Canned:		
Water pack, ½ cup		35
Syrup pack, ½ cup		90
Grapefruit juice:		
Raw, ½ cup		50
Canned:		
Unsweetened, ½ cup		50
Sweetened, ½ cup		65
Frozen concentrate, diluted, ready-to-serve:		
Unsweetened, ½ cup		50
Sweetened, ½ cup		60
Grapes, raw:		
American type (including Concord, Delaware, Niagara, and Scuppernong), slip skin, 1 bunch (½ × 3 inches; about 3½ ounces)		45
½ cup, with skins and seeds		30
European type (including Malaga, Muscat, Thompson seedless, and Flame Tokay, adherent skin), ½ cup		50

VEGETABLES AND FRUITS—Continued

Number of calories

Grape juice, bottled	½ cup	80
Honeydew melon, raw	1 wedge, 2 × 7 inches	50
Lemon juice, raw or canned	½ cup	30
	1 tablespoon	5
Lemonade, frozen concentrate, sweetened, diluted, ready-to-serve.	½ cup	55
Oranges, raw	1 orange, 3 inches in diameter.	75
Orange juice:		
Raw	½ cup	55
Canned, unsweetened	½ cup	60
Frozen concentrate, diluted, ready-to-serve.	½ cup	55
Peaches:		
Raw	1 medium, 2 inches in diameter (about ¼ pound).	35
	½ cup, sliced	30
Canned:		
Water pack	½ cup	40
Heavy syrup pack	½ cup	100
Dried, cooked, unsweetened.	½ cup (5 to 6 halves and 3 tablespoons syrup).	110
Frozen, sweetened	½ cup	105
Pears:		
Raw	1 pear, 3 × 2½ inches in diameter.	100
Canned in heavy syrup	½ cup	100
Pineapple:		
Raw	½ cup, diced	40
Canned in heavy syrup:		
Crushed	½ cup	100
Sliced	2 small or 1 large slice and 2 tablespoons juice.	90
Pineapple juice, canned	½ cup	70
Plums:		
Raw	1 plum, 2 inches in diameter (about 2 ounces).	25
Canned, syrup pack	½ cup	100
Prunes, dried, cooked:		
Unsweetened	½ cup (8 to 9 prunes and 2 tablespoons liquid).	150

Caloric Value of Selected Foods

VEGETABLES AND FRUITS—Continued

		Number of calories
Sweetened	½ cup (8 to 9 prunes and 2 tablespoons liquid).	255
Prune juice, canned	½ cup	100
Raisins, dried	½ cup	230
Rhubarb, cooked, sweetened	½ cup	190
Tangerine, raw	1 medium, 2½ inches in diameter (about ¼ pound).	40
Tangerine juice, canned	½ cup	50
Watermelon, raw	1 wedge, 4 × 8 inches long (about 2 pounds, including rind).	115

BREAD AND CEREALS

Bread:		
Cracked wheat	1 slice, ½ inch thick	60
Raisin	1 slice, ½ inch thick	60
Rye	1 slice, ½ inch thick	55
White	1 slice, ½ inch thick	60
Whole wheat	1 slice, ½ inch thick	55
Other baked goods:		
Baking powder biscuit	1 biscuit, 2½ inches in diameter.	140
Crackers:		
Graham	4 small or 2 medium	55
Saltines	2 crackers, 2 inches square	35
Soda	2 crackers, 2½ inches square	50
Oyster	10 crackers	45
Donuts (cake type)	1 donut	125
Muffins:		
Plain	1 muffin, 2¾ inches in diameter.	140
Bran	1 muffin, 2¾ inches in diameter.	130
Corn	1 muffin, 2¾ inches in diameter.	150
Pancakes (griddle cakes):		
Wheat (home recipe)	1 cake, 4 inches in diameter	60
Buckwheat (with buckwheat pancake mix).	1 cake, 4 inches in diameter	55
Pizza (cheese)	5½-inch sector, ⅛ of a 14-inch pie.	185

BREAD AND CEREALS—Continued

		Number of calories
Pretzels	5 small sticks	20
Rolls:		
Plain, pan	1 roll (16 ounces per dozen)	115
Hard, round	1 roll (22 ounces per dozen)	160
Sweet, pan	1 roll (18 ounces per dozen)	135
Rye wafers	2 wafers, 1⅞ × 3½ inches	45
Waffles	1 waffle, 4½ × 5½ inches × ½ inch.	210
Cereals and other grain products:		
Bran flakes (40-percent bran)	1 ounce (about ⅘ cup)	85
Corn, puffed, presweetened	1 ounce (about 1 cup)	110
Corn, shredded	1 ounce (about ⅘ cup)	110
Corn flakes	1 ounce (about 1⅓ cups)	110
Corn grits, degermed, cooked.	¾ cup	90
Farina, cooked	¾ cup	75
Macaroni, cooked	¾ cup	115
Macaroni and cheese	½ cup	235
Noodles, cooked	¾ cup	150
Oat cereal (mixture mainly oat flour).	1 ounce (about 1⅛ cups)	115
Oatmeal or rolled oats, cooked.	¾ cup	100
Rice, cooked	¾ cup	140
Rice flakes	1 cup (about 1 ounce)	115
Rice, puffed	1 cup (about ½ ounce)	55
Spaghetti, cooked	¾ cup	115
Spaghetti with meat balls	¾ cup	250
Spaghetti in tomato sauce, with cheese.	¾ cup	195
Wheat, puffed	1 ounce (about 2⅛ cups)	105
Wheat, puffed, presweetened.	1 ounce (about 2⅛ cups)	105
Wheat, rolled, cooked	¾ cup	130
Wheat, shredded, plain (long, round, or bite-size).	1 ounce (1 large biscuit or about ½ cup bite-size).	100
Wheat flakes	1 ounce (about ¾ cup)	100
Wheat flours:		
Whole wheat	¾ cup, stirred	300

BREAD AND CEREALS—Continued

		Number of calories
All-purpose (or family) flour.	¾ cup, sifted	300
Wheat germ	¾ cup, stirred	185

FATS, OILS, AND RELATED PRODUCTS

Butter or margarine	1 tablespoon	100
	1 pat or square (64 per pound).	50
Cooking fats:		
Vegetable	1 tablespoon	110
Lard	1 tablespoon	125
Salad or cooking oils	1 tablespoon	125
Salad dressings:		
French	1 tablespoon	60
Blue cheese, French	1 tablespoon	80
Home-cooked, boiled	1 tablespoon	30
Low-calorie	1 tablespoon	15
Mayonnaise	1 tablespoon	110
Salad dressing, commercial, plain (mayonnaise-type).	1 tablespoon	65
Thousand Island	1 tablespoon	75

DESSERTS

Apple betty	½ cup	170
Cakes:		
Angelcake	2-inch sector ($\frac{1}{12}$ of 8-inch round cake).	110
Butter cakes:		
Plain, without icing	1 piece, 3 × 2 × 1½ inches	200
	1 cupcake, 2¾ inches in diameter.	145
Plain, with chocolate icing.	2-inch sector ($\frac{1}{16}$ of 10-inch round layer cake).	370
	1 cupcake, 2¾ inches in diameter.	185
Chocolate, with chocolate icing.	2-inch sector ($\frac{1}{16}$ of 10-inch round layer cake).	445
Fruitcake, dark	1 piece, 2 × 2 × ½ inch.	115
Gingerbread	1 piece, 2 × 2 × 2 inches	175
Pound cake	1 slice, 2¾ × 3 × ⅝ inch.	140

DESSERTS—Continued

		Number of calories
Sponge cake	2-inch sector (1/12 of 8-inch round cake).	120
Cookies, plain and assorted	1 cookie, 3 inches in diameter.	120
Cornstarch pudding	½ cup	140
Custard, baked	½ cup	140
Figbars, small	1 figbar	55
Fruit ice	½ cup	75
Gelatin dessert, plain, ready-to-serve.	½ cup	70
Ice cream, plain	1 container (3½ fluid ounces).	130
Ice milk	½ cup (4 fluid ounces)	140
Pies:		
Apple	4-inch sector (1/7 of 9-inch pie).	345
Cherry	4-inch sector (1/7 of 9-inch pie).	355
Custard	4-inch sector (1/7 of 9-inch pie).	280
Lemon meringue	4-inch sector (1/7 of 9-inch pie).	305
Mince	4-inch sector (1/7 of 9-inch pie).	365
Pumpkin	4-inch sector (1/7 of 9-inch pie).	275
Prune whip	½ cup	105
Rennet dessert pudding, ready-to-serve.	½ cup	130
Sherbet	½ cup	130

SUGARS, SWEETS, AND RELATED PRODUCTS

Candy:		
Caramels	1 ounce (3 medium caramels).	115
Chocolate creams	1 ounce (2 to 3 pieces, 35 to a pound).	125
Chocolate, milk, sweetened	1-ounce bar	150
Chocolate, milk, sweetened with almonds.	1-ounce bar	150

Caloric Value of Selected Foods

SUGARS, SWEETS, AND RELATED PRODUCTS—Continued

Number of calories

Chocolate mints	1 ounce (1 to 2 pieces, 20 to a pound).	115
Fudge, milk chocolate, plain	1 ounce (1 piece, 1 to 1½ inches square).	115
Gumdrops	1 ounce (about 2½ large or 20 small).	100
Hard candy	1 ounce (3 to 4 candy balls, ¾ inch in diameter).	110
Jellybeans	1 ounce (10 beans)	105
Marshmallows	1 ounce (3 to 4 marshmallows, 60 to a pound).	90
Peanut brittle	1 ounce (1½ pieces, 2½ × 1¼ inches × ⅜ inch).	120
Syrup, honey, molasses:		
Chocolate syrup	1 tablespoon	50
Honey, strained or extracted	1 tablespoon	65
Molasses, cane, light	1 tablespoon	50
Syrup, table blends	1 tablespoon	60
Jelly	1 tablespoon	55
Jam, marmalade, preserves	1 tablespoon	55
Sugar: White, granulated, or brown.	1 teaspoon	15

SOUPS

Bean with pork	1 cup	170
Beef noodle	1 cup	70
Bouillon, broth, and consomme.	1 cup	30
Chicken noodle	1 cup	65
Clam chowder	1 cup	85
Cream of asparagus	1 cup	155
Cream of mushroom	1 cup	135
Minestrone	1 cup	105
Oyster stew	1 cup (3 to 4 oysters)	200
Tomato	1 cup	90
Vegetable with beef broth	1 cup	80

BEVERAGES (not including milk beverages and fruit juices)

Carbonated beverages:		
Ginger ale	8-ounce glass	70
Cola-type	8-ounce glass	95

BEVERAGES—Continued

		Number of calories
Alcoholic beverages:		
Beer, 3.6 percent alcohol by weight.	8-ounce glass	100
Whisky, gin, rum:		
100-proof	1 jigger (1½ ounces)	125
90-proof	1 jigger (1½ ounces)	110
86-proof	1 jigger (1½ ounces)	105
80-proof	1 jigger (1½ ounces)	100
70-proof	1 jigger (1½ ounces)	85
Wines:		
Table wines (such as Chablis, claret, Rhine wine, and sauterne).	1 wine glass (about 3 ounces).	75
Dessert wines (such as muscatel, port, sherry, and Tokay).	1 wine glass (about 3 ounces).	125

MISCELLANEOUS

Bouillon cube	1 cube, ⅝ inch	5
Olives:		
Green	4 medium or 3 extra large or 2 giant.	15
Ripe	3 small or 2 large	15
Pickles, cucumber:		
Dill	1 large, 1¾ inches in diameter × 4 inches long.	15
Sweet	1 pickle, ¾ inch in diameter × 2¾ inches long.	30
Popcorn, popped (with oil and salt added).	1 cup	65
Relishes and sauces:		
Chili sauce	1 tablespoon	20
Tomato catsup	1 tablespoon	15
Gravy	2 tablespoons	35
White sauce, medium (1 cup milk, 2 tablespoons fat, and 2 tablespoons flour).	½ cup	215
Cheese sauce (medium white sauce with 2 tablespoons cheese per cup).	½ cup	245

APPENDIX C

THE EQUATIONS GOVERNING WEIGHT CHANGE IN HUMAN BEINGS [*]

by Vincent Antonetti

The weight change in human beings resulting from a given diet is a function of at least the following parameters: age, sex, height, initial weight, amount of physical activity, caloric intake, changes in body hydration, and the duration of the diet. Due to the many factors involved, it is thus difficult to predict accurately what weight change to expect for an individual on a known diet during a given period of time. Nevertheless, several reports in the literature ranging from Benedict (1) to Forbes (2), have proposed mathematical expressions devised to predict weight loss as a function of time. The approach taken in these reports was to fit a mathematical equation to observed empirical data. However, most of the important parameters previously mentioned were not considered.

This paper takes an engineering approach to the analysis of the problem of weight change in human beings. First, a thermodynamic energy balance is used to relate pertinent variables in equation form. Next, data published in the literature

---

[*] Reprinted from The American Journal of Clinical Nutrition, Vol. 26, No. 1, January, 1973.

Nomenclature: A, surface area, ft^2; B, basal metabolic rate, kcal/hour meter^2; C, kcal/day; d, (derivative); E, energy, kcal; E' energy, kcal/day; H, height, inches; K_A, activity coefficient, kcal/lb/day; K_B, basal metabolic coefficient, kcal/lb/day; Q, heat loss, kcal; U, internal energy, kcal; W, weight, lb; W_k, work, kcal; α, allowance for specific dynamic action, dimensionless fraction; Θ, time, days; γ, energy value of body weight lost or gained.

Subscripts: A, activity; B, basal; D, diet; f, final or food; L, loss; o, initial w, waste.

are used to deduce needed coefficients. Then, the basic differential equation developed is solved using numerical integration methods. The result is an analytical technique that can be used to predict weight change as a function of time for an individual on any known diet. In addition, the theory developed is checked and found to agree quite well with clinical data.

Analysis

The human body may be represented thermodynamically by the closed system pictured in Fig. 1. Applying the principle

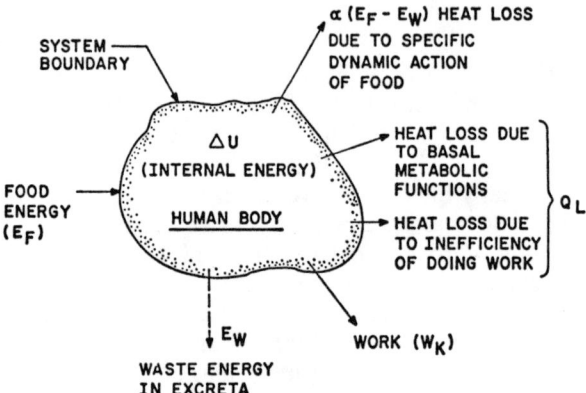

FIG. 1. Thermodynamic representation of the human body.

of the conservation of energy, the change in the internal energy (ΔU) of the system during the time interval ($\Delta \Theta$) is equal to the difference between the total energy entering and leaving the system boundaries during this period of time (3). Therefore, the general energy equation for the system may be written as:

$$\Delta U = (1 - \alpha)(E_f - E_w) - (Q_L + W_k) \qquad (1)$$

where α is an allowance for the specific dynamic action of food.

Now define the net caloric value of food per unit of time as $C_D = (E_f - E_w)/\Delta \Theta$, and the calories per unit of time required to offset heat lost to the ambient plus any work performed as $C = (Q_L + W_k)/\Delta\Theta$. Then, after substitution and rearrangement equation 1 becomes:

$$\frac{\Delta U}{\Delta\Theta} = (1-\alpha)C_D - C \qquad (2)$$

It is well known that energy and mass are mutually convertible, and that physiologically, when there is a discrepancy between caloric intake and expenditure, a change in body weight occurs. This principle allows the change in internal energy to be expressed as a change in weight (ΔW) multiplied by a constant of proportionality (γ). For very small changes in the system ($\Delta W/\Delta\Theta$) = ($dW/d\Theta$), the resulting equation may be expressed in differential form as:

$$\frac{dW}{d\Theta} = \frac{(1-\alpha)C_D - C}{\gamma} \qquad (3)$$

Equation 3 given above states that the change in body weight with respect to time ($dW/d\Theta$) is equal to the caloric value of the food consumed, minus the calories needed to maintain a particular weight, all divided by γ which is the energy value, per unit of weight, of body mass lost or gained during caloric imbalance. The value sometimes used in the literature as an approximation for γ is 3,500 kcal/lb. This analysis makes the simplifying assumption that γ is constant during weight changes, although it has been shown by Brožek et al. (4) that this is not the case.

In order to develop the analysis further, an expression for the energy expenditure (C) is needed.* This parameter may be thought of as the sum of two functions: an activity energy function (E'_A) and a basal metabolic energy function (E'_B). Stated algebraically, this reads:

$$C = E'_A + E'_B \qquad (4)$$

* As the energy requirements for growth in children seem to be less understood than the weight gain process for adults, this analysis will be restricted to adults. The analysis also assumes that the amount of fluid entering the body equals the amount leaving. Whereas this assumption may not be valid for short time increments, it should apply in the long run.

The activity energy (E'_A) is directly proportional to the body weight:

$$E'_A = K_A W \qquad (5)$$

In this paper, K_A, a constant of proportionality, will be called the activity coefficient.

The activity coefficient K_A is the sum of the calories expended per pound of body weight for each activity, multiplied by the time spent at each activity.

Because such a detailed calculation will for most individuals be impractical, Taylor and Pye (5) have suggested a short method that is adopted for use in this paper. Essentially, this short method lists calories expended per pound per hour for various degrees of activity, ranging from persons at rest to those engaged in severe exercise. K_A was computed from the values (5) by assuming 16 active hours per day. Therefore, the units of K_A are calories per pound per day. Table 1 lists values of K_A determined in this manner.

TABLE 1

Values of activity coefficient (K_A)[a]

Level of activity	K_B (kcal/lb/day)
Sedentary	3.68
Light	4.32
Moderate	5.75
Vigorous	8.00
Severe	12.30

[a] These values were derived from data shown in (5).

The other component of the energy expenditure equation is the basal metabolic energy.

Essentially, there are two schools of thought regarding what method to use when describing the basal metabolic energy E'_B. The first method assumes that E'_B is proportional to the body surface area. The second method considers E'_B to be proportional to the body weight to a fractional power.

If the surface area approach is used, as in the first method, then E'_B is directly proportional to the basal metabolic rate (B) and the surface area (A). Using an expression for the surface area suggested by DuBois (6) and converting the units of the equation to the English system of pounds and inches, the basal metabolic energy for a 24-hr period can be shown as:

$$E'_B = 0.241(B)(H^{0.725})(W^{0.425}).$$

Now define $K_B = 0.241(B)(H^{0.725})$, and the expression for the basal metabolic energy can be stated as:

$$E'_B = K_B W^{0.425} \qquad (6)$$

If, however, as stated in the second method, the body weight to a fractional power is employed, the E'_B can be expressed as (7):

$$E'_B = K_B W^{0.73} \qquad (6A)$$

If each of the two methods is considered separately, then the value of the basal metabolic coefficient K_B is also different for each case, as shown in equations 6 and 6A. In the case in which the surface area law is used (equation 6), K_B is a function of sex, age, and height; in equation 6A, however, K_B is a function of only sex and age.

To incorporate both methods of expressing the basal metabolic energy and also to continue the analysis in the most general manner, the basal metabolic energy is expressed as:

$$E'_B = K_B W^n \qquad (6B)$$

where: $n = 0.425$ for the surface area approach, and
$n = 0.73$ for the body weight approach
and values of K_B for both techniques are listed in Table 2.

Now the expressions for the activity energy (E'_A) and the basal metabolic energy (E'_B), described by equations 5 and 6B, respectively, are substituted in equation 4 to yield:

$$C = K_A W + K_B W^n \qquad (7)$$

During steady-state conditions when the amount of calories consumed equals the amount required to offset total maintenance requirements, equation 7 may be converted to what will be called the "weight maintenance equation" by noting

TABLE 2

Values of basal metabolic coefficient (K_B) [a]
Surface area method: $K_B = E'_B/W^{0.425} = 0.241 (B)(H)^{0.725}$

		Height, inches		
Sex	Age	60 to 66	66 to 72	72 to 78
Male	18–35	186	199	210
	35–55	175.7	183.5	199
	55–75	164	171.5	186
Female	18–35	180	182	192
	35–55	164	171.5	186
	55–75	154.5	162	175

[a] Average values for B were obtained from (11–13).

Weight method: $K_B = E'_B/W^{0.73}$

Sex	Age	K_B
Male	18–35	43
	35–55	40.6
	55–75	38
Female	18–35	39.2
	35–55	38
	55–75	35.9

that α calories consumed will be lost as heat due to specific dynamic action. This done, equation 7 becomes:

$$C = \frac{1}{(1-\alpha)}(K_A W + K_B W^n) \qquad (8)$$

Equation 8 is used to determine the caloric intake needed, by an adult of given sex, age, height, and activity level, to maintain a particular weight.

Continuing the analysis, the expression for the caloric intake (C) from equation 7 is now substituted into equation 3. The result is:

$$\frac{dW}{d\theta} = \frac{(1-\alpha)C_D - (K_A W + K_B W^n)}{\gamma}.$$

This differential equation may be solved by separating variables and integrating:

$$\theta = \gamma \int_{W_0}^{W_f} \frac{dW}{(1-\alpha)C_D - (K_A W + K_B W^n)} \quad (9)$$

However, the exponent n makes an explicit solution difficult. For this reason, a numerical integration technique known as Simpson's Rule (8) is used to arrive at an answer. In this technique, the solution of equation 9 is the following formula:

$$\theta = \frac{\gamma(W_f - W_0)}{3p} \quad (10)$$

$$[f_0 + 4f_1 + 2f_2 + 4f_3 + \cdots 2f_{p-2} + 4f_{p-1} + f_p]$$

where p = number of integration intervals chosen (p = 4, 6, 8, 10, et cetera), although p should be large enough to assure the integration will be accurate. This writer has found that solutions are quite accurate if p = 10.

The individual functions f_0, f_1, f_2, et cetera, are defined as:

$$f_j = [(1-\alpha)C_D - (K_A W_j + K_B W_j^n)]^{-1} \quad (11)$$

where,

$$W_j = W_0 - \frac{j}{p}(W_0 - W_f), \quad j = 0 \text{ to } p \quad (12)$$

The calculation technique using the derived equations given above is illustrated by the following examples.

Example 1: Using equation 8, determine the caloric allowance for the so-called "Reference Man" and "Reference Woman." Let n = 0.425 (surface area law assumed for this calculation).

A) Reference Man is defined (9) as being 22 years of age, 154 lb, and 69 inches tall. His activity level is described as moderate. Therefore, from Table 1, K_A = 5.75 kcal/lb per day and from Table 2, $K_B = 199$ kcal/lb per day. Let $\alpha = 0.1$ (10% allowance for specific dynamic action). Then, the caloric intake required to maintain 154 lb is determined by equation 8 as:

$$C = 1.11(K_A W + K_B W^{0.425})$$
$$= 1.11(5.75(154) + 199(154)^{0.425})$$
$$= 2{,}830 \text{ kcal/day}$$

This is in close agreement with the given value of 2,800 kcal/day (9).

B) Reference Woman is defined as being 22 years of age, 128 lb, and 64 inches tall. Her activity level is close to what in this paper is called light. Therefore, $K_A = 4.32$ and $K_B = 170$. Then, the caloric intake required to maintain 128 lb is $C = 1.1 \ (4.32(128) + 170(128)^{0.425}) = 2{,}070$ kcal/day. This is within 4% of the value of 2,000 kcal/day (9).

Example 2: How long will it take a 30-year-old male, 63 inches tall and 180 lb to lose 50 lb on a diet of 2,100 kcal/day? Assume his activity level can be described as light and $n = 0.425$ (surface area law applies).

From Table 1, $K_A = 4.32$ and from Table 2, $K_B = 186$. Though not necessary for the solution, it is interesting to calculate this individual's caloric intake at 180 lb. Using equation 8 and the procedure illustrated in example 1, the maintenance calories are found to be 2,715 kcal/day. The amount of time to lose 50 lb can now be calculated.

For purposes of comparison, we will look first at the calculation technique oftentimes referred to in the literature (10) as the "classical method" and then at the new "proposed method" that the author has developed.

A. *Classical method.* Using equation 7, the amount of energy intake needed to sustain 180 lb (exclusive of specific dynamic action) is found to be 2,470 kcal/day. The difference between energy intake and expenditure is then computed $(2{,}470 - (2{,}100 - 210)) = 580$ kcal/day. Note here that 10% was allowed for specific dynamic action. The time to lose 50 lb is calculated as:

$$\theta = \frac{3{,}500(50)}{580} = 302 \text{ days}$$

B. *Proposed method.* Equation 10 is used with $\gamma = 3{,}500$, $\alpha = 0.10$, and $p = 10$. The sum of the individual functions

f_0, f_1 to f_{10} can be shown to be -0.09345. The time to lose 50 lb is then:

$$\theta = \frac{\gamma(W_f - W_0)}{3p}[f_0 + 4f_1 + \cdots + f_p]$$

$$\theta = \frac{3{,}500(130-180)}{3(10)}[-0.09345] = 545 \text{ days}$$

Comparing the answers arrived at using the two different approaches, it can be seen that for this example, the use of the classical method results in an error of almost 50%.

Because of this substantial error, a discussion of the main difference between the classical method and the analytical technique presented in this paper is in order at this time.

As an individual loses weight, his maintenance caloric requirements decrease with time. This is a fundamental concept which the classical method does not take into account. For instance, the subject in example 2 required 2,715 kcal/day for maintenance at the start of the diet when his body weight was 180 lb, but needed only 2,430 kcal/day for maintenance after his body weight had fallen to 150 lb, et cetera. The analytical technique proposed in this paper takes this aspect into account whereas the classical method does not. This then is the key difference between the two methods.

The error between the classical and proposed solutions increases as the diet calories approach that required to sustain the desired final body weight. For instance, for the subject in this example, a caloric intake of 2,100 kcal/day can be shown via equation 8 as sufficient to sustain a body weight of 120 lb. Therefore, if a weight loss of 60 lb is desired on this diet, it should require theoretically an infinite amount of time. This is shown graphically in Fig. 2. The curvilinear shape of the weight loss curve agrees with several reports in the literature, for example Forbes (2), which have suggested that weight loss is exponential in nature.

Further questions may be asked. How would the weight loss curve be altered if the diet were 1,200 kcal/day? What is the effect of increased activity? Whereas the numerical calculation technique proposed is time-consuming when performed by hand, the procedure, however, is easily programmed for a digital computer. This done, sufficient data points are made

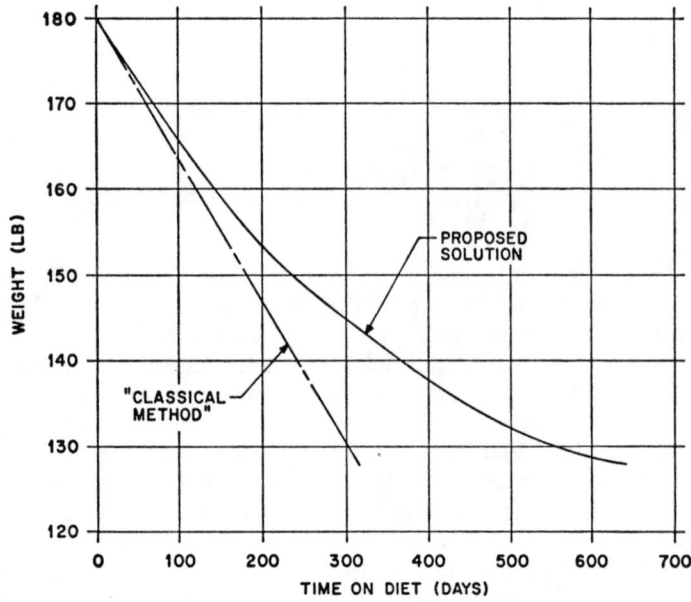

Fig. 2. Weight versus time for subject in example 2.

available to answer the questions posed. Figure 3 shows the effect of diet, whereas Fig. 4 presents the effect of activity.

Comparison of theory with clinical data

In this section, the analytical predictions of equation 10 will be compared with clinical observations. Although there is a great deal of data available, a large segment of the published reports is not sufficiently complete with regard to age, height, activity level, et cetera, to provide a valid test for equation 10.

After a review of the literature, it was decided to compare equation 10 with the data of Keys et al. (14). However, even in this well-documented treatise, there is a question as to the manner and extent of the subjects' decrease in spontaneous activity. I was able to deduce the mean activity coefficient (K_A) of the subjects at the start and end of the experiment from the data presented in a follow-up paper by Taylor and Keys (15). Figure 5 shows the prediction of the weight loss curve made using equation 10 compared with the mean data for the group of 32 subjects of the Minnesota experiment. The

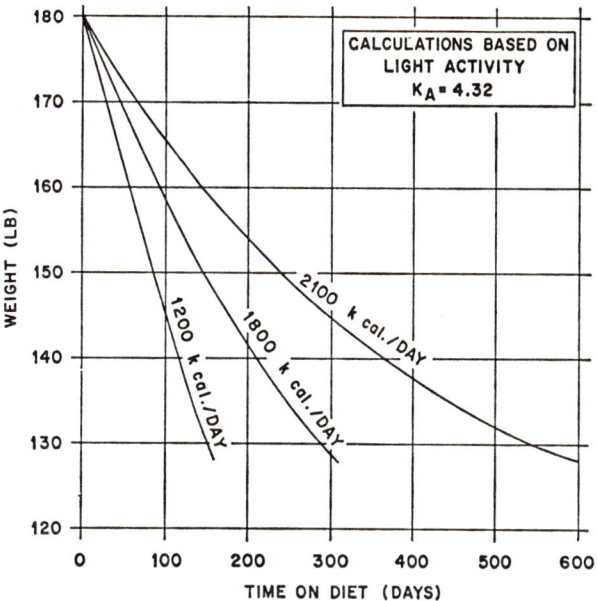

Fig. 3. Weight loss curves for subject in example 2 illustrating the effect of diet.

surface area form of equation 10 (n = 0.425) was employed in addition to the assumptions for K_A noted in Fig 5. As can be seen from Fig. 5, equation 10 agrees quite well with the data except for the last few weeks. The deviation between theory and data can be attributed to the fact that most of the subjects suffered from famine edema toward the end of the experiment.

In order to limit the number of assumptions required, particularly with regard to activity level and caloric intake, it was decided to check equation 10 for a fasting patient confined to a hospital. Figure 6 shows the prediction of equation 10 as compared with the well-documented data of Gilder et al. (16). It appears, for the patient shown, that equation 10, based on the surface area approach, comes closer to the experimental data than when the body weight approach (n = 0.73) is used. This is merely an observation, and it is not implied that this will be true in all situations.

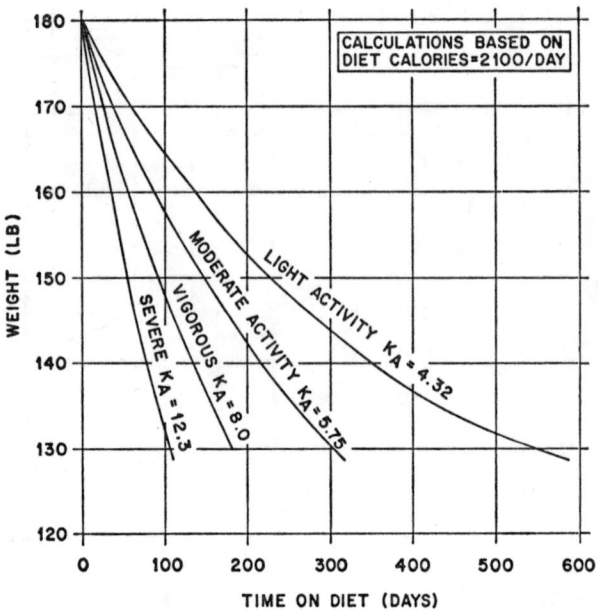

Fig. 4. Weight loss curves for subject in example 2 illustrating the effect of various activity levels.

The preceding comparisons were limited to a small sample of the published data, and of course, are not sufficient to conclusively prove the validity of the weight loss equation derived in this paper. Further comparisons with observed data should be made. This author, however, feels that a more detailed study should be the subject of a follow-up paper, more properly written by researchers with more access to the data.

Limitations

The most general approach to solve the current problem would be to relate all the variables in the exact manner that they affect the physical problem. However, this is not always practical, and in this paper, several simplifying assumptions were made in order that the resulting mathematics be manageable. It should therefore be noted that the use of the weight change equation derived in this paper is constrained by the fact that the caloric equivalent of weight loss (γ), the

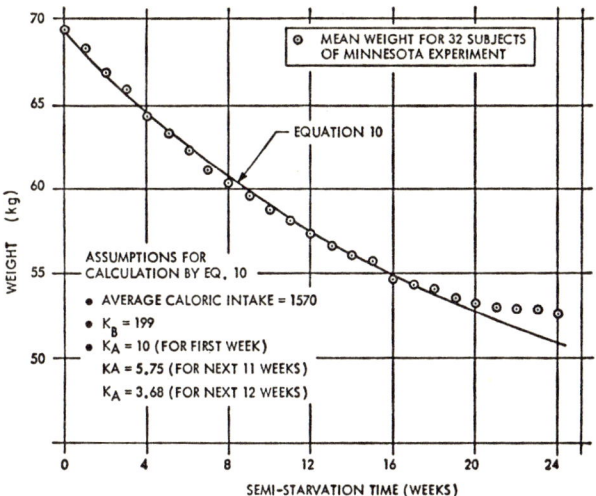

Fig. 5. Comparison of theory with Minnesota experiment of Keys et al. (14).

basal metabolic rate, and the activity level coefficient (K_A) were assumed to be constant during weight change.

It is well known that body mass changes during energy deficit are of variable composition. Fat, water, and protein are lost at different rates at different times. Energy value of body weight lost will be low during the first few days of caloric deficit due to the considerable loss of water. It is reasonable therefore to expect that assuming γ to be constant would be most inaccurate during short periods of energy imbalance.

One of the adaptive factors during weight loss is a decrease in the basal metabolic rate in negative energy balance. According to Grande et al. (17), it seems possible that the decrease in basal metabolic rate does not progress after a certain time. Therefore, the assumption that the basal metabolic rate is constant with time should become less significant as the duration of the diet increases.

Another adaptive response to calorie restriction is a decrease in the level of spontaneous activity (K_A). This fact probably would not be important for the obese individual reducing to a more normal weight at moderate calorie deficits. However,

276 The Computer Diet

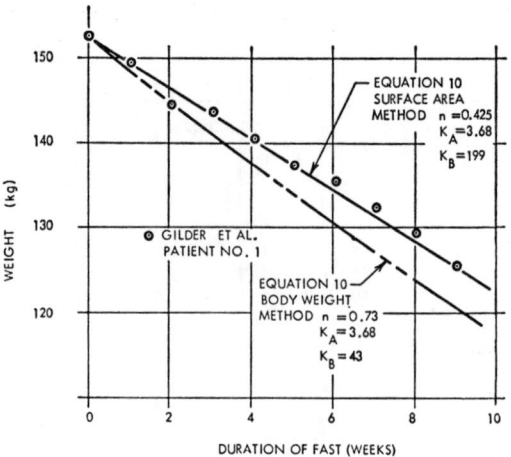

FIG. 6. Comparison of theory with data of Gilder et al. (16).

for the person subjected to a semistarvation diet, this factor is important and must be taken into account. Changes in activity level can be accounted for if anticipated when the calculation using equation 10 is performed. If the decrease in activity level can be quantitatively stated as a function of weight or time, then equation 9 can be solved by a procedure called stepwise integration. In fact, this was the technique employed to calculate the curve labeled equation 10 for the Minnesota experiment shown in Fig. 5.

Just how limiting the preceding factors are will only be determined after the proposed weight loss equation is compared with considerably more observed data.

Summary

Two useful and basic equations have been derived. Equation 8 can be used to calculate the caloric intake per day required to maintain a particular weight level. Equation 10 can be used to calculate weight change as a function of time for a particular caloric intake. Tables 1 and 2 list values of coefficients K_A and K_B and are utilized in conjunction with equations 8 and 10.

It may be difficult in some cases to assume a constant caloric intake, and, in particular, to predict accurately the activity level. However, even in instances when exact values of the variables cannot be determined with confidence, equation 10 can be utilized to compute the range and trends of the weight loss as a function of all pertinent parameters (similar to Figs. 3 and 4). A further value of equation 10 is its organizing effect in the study of the many variables involved in weight change.

References

1. BENEDICT, F. G. *A Study of Prolonged Fasting.* Carnegie Inst. Publ. No. 203, Washington, D.C., 1915.
2. FORBES, G. B. Weight loss during fasting: implications for the obese. *Am. J. Clin. Nutr.* 23:1212, 1970.
3. ZEMANSKY, M. W. *Heat and Thermodynamics.* New York: McGraw-Hill, 1957, p. 61.
4. BROŽEK, J., F. GRANDE, H. L. TAYLOR, J. T. ANDERSON, E. R. BUSKIRK AND A. KEYS. Changes in body weight and body dimensions in men performing work on a low calorie carbohydrate diet. *J. Appl. Physiol.* 10:412, 1957.
5. TAYLOR, C. M., AND O. F. PYE. *Foundations of Nutrition.* New York: Macmillan, 1966, p. 48.
6. DUBOIS, E. F. *Basal Metabolism in Health and Disease.* Philadelphia: Lea & Febiger, 1936, p. 494.
7. Food and Agriculture Organization of the United Nations. *FAO Nutrition Study No. 15,* Rome, 1965, p. 19.
8. SALVADORI, M. G., AND M. L. BARON. *Numerical Methods in Engineering.* New Jersey: Prentice-Hall, 1959, p. 72.
9. Recommended Dietary Allowances. *Natl. Acad. Sci.—Natl. Res. Council Publ.* No. 1694, Washington, D.C., 1968.
10. BRAY, G. A. The myth of diet in the management of obesity. *Am. J. Clin. Nutr.* 23:1141, 1970.
11. BOOTHBY, W. M., J. BERKSON AND H. L. DUNN. Studies of the energy of metabolism of normal individuals: a standard for basal metabolism, with a nomogram for clinical applications. *Am. J. Physiol.* 116:468, 1936.
12. BERKSON, J., AND W. M. BOOTHBY. Studies of the energy of metabolism of normal individuals. A comparison of the estimation of basal metabolism from (1) a linear formula and (2) "surface area." *Am. J. Physiol.* 116:485, 1936.
13. BERKSON, J., AND W. M. BOOTHBY. Studies of the energy of metabolism of normal individuals. *Am. J. Physiol.* 121: 669, 1938.
14. KEYS, A., J. BROŽEK, A. HENSCHEL, O. MICKELSEN AND H. L. TAYLOR. *Biology of Human Starvation.* Minneapolis: Univ. of Minnesota Press, 1950, vol. 2, p. 1128.
15. TAYLOR, H. L., AND A. KEYS. Adaptation to caloric restriction. *Science* 112:215, 1950.

16. GILDER, H., G. N. CORNELL, W. R. GRAFE, J. R. MACFARLANE, J. W. ASAPH, W. T. STUBENBORD, G. M. WATKINS, J. R. REES AND B. THORBJARNARSON. Components of weight loss in obese patients subjected to prolonged starvation. *J. Appl. Physiol.* 23: 304, 1967.
17. GRANDE, F., J. T. ANDERSON AND A. KEYS. Changes in basal metabolic rate in man in semistarvation and refeeding. *J. Appl. Physiol.* 12:230, 1958.

APPENDIX D

BIBLIOGRAPHY

Chapter 1

Antonetti, V. W. "The equations governing weight change in human beings." *Am. J. Clin. Nutr.* 26:64, 1973.

Atwater, W. O. and Benedict, F. G. "Experiments on the metabolism of matter and energy in the human body." *U.S. Dept. Agriculture Exptl. Sta. Bull.* 136, 1903.

Bray, G. A. "The myth of diet in the management of obesity." *Am. J. Clin. Nutr.* 23:1141, 1970.

Fan, L. T., Hsu, F. T., and Hwang, C. L. "A review of mathematical models of the human thermal system." IEEE Transactions on Bio-Medical Engineering Vol. *BME*-18, No. 3, May 1971.

Keys, A., Brozek, J., Henschel, A., Mickalsen, O., and Taylor, H. L. *Biology of Human Starvation.* Univ. of Minnesota Press, Vol. 1, 1950.

Kinsell, L. W., Gunning, B., Michaels, G. P., Richardson, J., and Cox, S. E. "Calories do count" *Metab. Clin. Expte.* 13:195, 1964.

Newburgh, L. H. *Physiology of Heat Regulation.* Hafner Publishing Co., New York, 1968.

Rombach, J. "Metabolic balance analysis program." COSMIC program documentation, Univ. of Georgia, 1970.

Thermal Problems in Biotechnology. Symposium of American Society of Mechanical Engineers, 1968.

Werner, S. C. "Comparison between weight reduction on a high calorie, high fat diet and on an isocaloric regime high in carbohydrates." *New Engl. J. Med.* 252:661, 1955.

Zemansky, M. W. *Heat and Thermodynamics.* McGraw-Hill, New York, 1957.

Chapter 2

Brody, S. *Bioenergetics and Growth*. Rheinhold, New York, 1945.

Grande, F. "Energetics and Weight Reduction." *Amer. J. Clin. Nutr.* 21:305, 1968.

Grollman, S. *The Human Body*. MacMillan, New York, 1964.

Kleiber, M. *The Fire of Life*. John Wiley, New York, 1961.

Lehniger, A. L. *Bioenergetics*. Benjamin, New York, 1965.

Morrison, T. F., Cornett, F. D., and Tether, J. E. *Human Physiology*. Holt, Rinehart and Winston, Inc., New York, 1963.

Chapter 3

Cooper, K. H. *Aerobics*. M. Evans and Co. Inc., New York, 1968.

Davis, A. *Let's Eat Right to Keep Fit*. New American Library, New York, 1970.

Kraus, B. *Calories and Carbohydrates*. Grosset and Dunlap, New York, 1971.

McHenry, E. W. *Basic Nutrition*. J. B. Lippincott, Philadelphia, 1973.

Nasset, E. S. *Your Diet, Digestion and Health*. Barnes and Noble, New York, 1962.

National Research Council, *Recommended Dietary Allowances*. Publication No. 1694, Washington, D.C., 1968.

Rosakamm, H. "Optimum patterns of exercise for healthy adults." *J. Canadian Med. Assoc.* 96:150, 1967.

Royal Canadian Air Force Exercise Plan for Physical Fitness. Pocket Books Inc., Canada, 1962.

Taylor, C. M., and Pye, O. F. *Foundations of Nutrition*. MacMillan, New York, 1966.

U.S. Department of Agriculture Home and Garden Bulletin No. 1. "Family fare: a guide to good nutrition." Washington, D.C., 1970.

U.S. Dept. of Agriculture Home and Garden Bulletin No. 72, "Nutritive Value of Foods." Washington, D.C., 1971.

Chapter 4

Glennon, J. A. "Weight reduction—an enigma." *Arch. Internal Med.* 118:1, 1966.

Jordan, H. A. "In defense of body weight." *J. Am. Dietetic Assoc.* 62:17, 1973.

U.S. Department of Agriculture Home and Garden Bulletin No. 74. "Food and your weight." Washington, D.C., 1969.

Van Itallie, T. B. and Campbell, R. G. "Multidisciplinary approach to obesity." *J. Am. Dietetic Assoc.* 61:385, 1972.

Chapter 5

Brožek, J., Grande, F., Taylor, H. L., Anderson, T. J., Buskirk, E. R., and Keys, A. "Changes in body weight and dimensions in men performing work on a low-calorie carbohydrate diet." *J. Appl. Physiol.* 10:412, 1957.

Buskirk, E. R., Thompson, R. H., Lutwak, L. and Whedon, G. D. "Energy balance of obese patients during weight reduction: influence of diet restrictions and exercise." *Ann. N.Y. Acad. Sci.* 110:918, 1963.

Gamble, J. L. *Companionship of Water and Electrolytes in the Organization of Body Fluids.* (Lane Medical Lectures) Stanford Univ. Press, 1951.

Chapter 6

Chaney, M. S. and Ross, M. L. *Nutrition.* Houghton Mifflin Company, Boston, 1966.

U.S. Dept. of Agriculture Home and Garden Bulletin No. 72, "Nutritive Values of Foods." Washington, D.C., 1971.

Chapter 7

Lamb, L. E. *Your Heart and How to Live With It.* Viking Press, New York, 1969.

Mayer, J. *Overweight: Causes, Cost and Control.* Prentice-Hall, New Jersey, 1968.

Chapter 8

Miller, D. S., Mumford, P., and Stock, M. J. "Gluttony 2: Thermogenesis in overeating man." *Am. J. Clin. Nutr.* 20:1223, 1967.

Stunkard, A., and McLaren-Hume, M. "The results of treatment for obesity." *Arch. Internal Med.* 103:79, 1959.

Chapter 9

Claiborne, C. *The New York Times Cookbook.* Harper and Row, New York, 1961.

McWilliams, M. *Food Fundamentals.* John Wiley and Sons, Inc., New York, 1966.

U.S. Dept. of Agriculture Home and Garden Bulletin No. 72, "Nutritive Value of Foods." Washington, D.C., 1971.

Chapter 10

Carlson, A. J., Johnson, V., and Cavert, H. M. *The Machinery of the Body*. Univ. Chicago Press, 1961.

Jolliffe, N. *Reduce and Stay Reduced.* Simon and Schuster, New York, 1963.